Thinner Leaner Stronger Cookbook

Flavors of Health, Exploring Diet through Meal Plans, Recipes, and Expert Methods

Tamara Chandler

Table Of Content

INTRODUCTION

How can we attain the desired trifecta of being "Thinner, Leaner, and Stronger" amid the hustle and bustle of contemporary life, when time is as valuable as gold and our plates are typically loaded with convenience over nutrition?

Take a minute to imagine...

You don't have the luxury of spending all your time in the gym since you aren't an outstanding athlete. A symphony of meetings, due dates, and obligations fills your day. But you secretly wish you were a healthier, more energetic version of yourself. You want to get rid of the additional weight, build lean muscle, and generate an abundance of energy that permeates every action you do.

Numerous people who have started on this trip report that it often starts with high goals and spectacular promises. However, somewhere along the line, such goals may get buried by the difficulties of daily existence. Have we not all been there?

What if I told you that there is a culinary compass that may help you in your search for health and vitality? Would it give you any reason for hope? Please enjoy your visit to the "Thinner Leaner Stronger Cookbook: Flavors of Health."

This is not just another cookbook; it is your dependable ally in your quest for better health. This cookbook is a game-changer for fitness fanatics, health-conscious readers, and anybody looking to make a permanent lifestyle shift. It has the same philosophical foundation as the well-known "Thinner Leaner Stronger" program, which has changed countless lives all over the globe.

Here, we lead you on a gastronomic journey where "health" and "delicious" live in peace. Our recipes are more than simply meals; they are your go-to tools for achieving your fitness objectives. Whether you're a regular gym goer, a busy professional, an aspiring athlete, or just someone ready to embrace a life teeming with well-being, we've deliberately prepared this cookbook with you in mind.

You'll discover a wealth of delectable recipes in these pages, all of which are intended to fuel your body, titillate your taste buds, and get you one step closer to your goal of becoming fitter, leaner, and stronger. That's not all, however. We simplify the science behind balanced nutrition, provide you with knowledge about meal planning, and show you how to cook in a way that will make you feel like a gourmet master.

You will read about real people, just like you, who have undergone amazing changes thanks to the information and dishes in this cookbook as we travel together through these pages. These experiences are proof of the value of taking charge of your nutrition and making it a key component of your quest for health and fitness.

Are you prepared to open the doors to a healthier version of yourself, one delectable meal at a time? You are invited to go on a gastronomic trip with the "Thinner Leaner Stronger Cookbook: Flavors of Health" that will change the way you see food, exercise, and ultimately, yourself. This voyage is one that should be enjoyed, and it starts here, in these pages.

Welcome to your path toward a better lifestyle and a more powerful, energetic self. We are here to lead you along a road that is founded in the age-old understanding of balanced nutrition in a society that is overrun with dietary fads and short cures. Your culinary companion, this cookbook has been painstakingly designed to perfectly integrate with the tenets of the well-known "Thinner Leaner Stronger" program.

The key to any successful fitness regimen is a balanced diet. It's not simply about calculating calories or giving up your favorite tastes; it's about intentionally fueling your body while relishing each mouthful. This cookbook will be your reliable ally whether you're starting your first fitness journey or want to optimize your dietary strategy.

You'll find a treasure mine of recipes intended to satisfy your appetite and inspire your goals in the pages that follow. We'll go into the science-backed approaches that support the "Thinner Leaner Stronger" mindset as well as the art of meal planning and portion management. Each dish is a gourmet celebration of health that has been thoughtfully created to support your fitness objectives without compromising taste or pleasure.

You'll discover that we've eliminated the element of guessing from meal planning as you browse through these recipes. We've thoughtfully selected a wide variety of foods to meet your requirements, from invigorating breakfasts to filling dinners and guilt-free snacks. Our customized meal plans will serve as your guide whether your goal is to lose weight, gain muscle, or just maintain a healthy lifestyle.

So, flip the page and enter a world where wellness is a way of life if you're ready to set out on a journey where health meets taste and exercise meets sustenance. Together, we'll investigate the "Flavors of Health" and learn how conscious, enjoyable eating may help you achieve your fitness goals.

Chapter 1

The Foundations of a Leaner, Stronger You

Achieving a leaner, stronger body might seem like a distant goal in the fast-paced world of today. We may feel overwhelmed and bewildered by the never-ending sea of diet fads, exercise fads, and contradicting advice. It doesn't have to be this way, however. Welcome to the "Thinner Leaner Stronger Cookbook," a transforming journey where we'll set out to learn the fundamentals of a healthier, more energetic you.

The Thinner Leaner Stronger Approach Revealed

The Thinner Leaner Stronger method of exercise sits at the center of our journey. Numerous people have been helped by this well-known method, created by fitness guru Michael Matthews, to not only lose extra weight but also develop long-lasting strength and energy. It is a system that is founded on science, supported by years of study, and refined by examples of real-world success.

The primary tenet of Thinner Leaner Stronger is the achievement of long-lasting effects via sustainable, research-based methods. We'll discuss how crucial it is to establish reasonable objectives, monitor your progress, and make use of the strength of consistency and discipline. This method recognizes that exercise is a lifetime commitment to your health, not simply a temporary pursuit.

What Makes a Balanced Diet?

Understanding the essential elements of a balanced diet is crucial as you set out on your road to a leaner, stronger self. We'll look at the vital nutrients your body needs to function, from vitamins and minerals to macronutrients like proteins, lipids, and carbs. You'll learn how these components interact to improve your metabolism, increase your energy, and assist the development and recuperation of your muscles.

However, this goes beyond sterile nutritional theory. Throughout this book, we'll demonstrate how to use this knowledge to prepare delicious meals that will satisfy your appetite and provide you energy. We are here to show that healthy eating can be a voyage of gastronomic joy. No more boring diets or restricted eating programs.

The Function of Meal Preparation and Cooking

Meal preparation and cooking are your most powerful partners in the fight for a leaner, more powerful self. They give you the authority to take charge of your nutrition, modify your meals in accordance with your precise objectives, and enjoy the tastes of health. This book will provide you with the knowledge and techniques required to master the art of cooking wholesome, delectable meals, whether you're a newbie in the kitchen or an experienced chef.

Learn the tricks of effective meal preparation so you may save time and effort while still achieving your fitness objectives. You'll learn how to maneuver the kitchen with assurance and creativity, from organizing your weekly meals to choosing the freshest ingredients. Each recipe includes a list of ingredients, step-by-step directions, and a nutritional analysis, making it simple to keep track of your consumption and make wise decisions.

To become a slimmer, stronger version of yourself, remember that life transformation, not just physical change, is what it takes. You'll not only find the way to your fitness objectives with the Thinner Leaner Stronger Cookbook as your guide, but you'll also get to experience the pleasures of delicious, healthy food. Let's start this thrilling journey toward a better version of ourselves, one delectable meal at a time.

Chapter 2

Laying the Groundwork - Simple Meal Planning

Meal planning is a potent tool that may be the difference between success and stagnation in your quest for a leaner, stronger self. To attain your fitness objectives, it's important to deliberately fuel your body in addition to what you consume. We will go deeply into the art and science of meal planning in this chapter, breaking it down into manageable parts.

Knowing Macronutrients and How They Play a Part in Your Diet

Let's take a trip to understand macronutrients, the cornerstone of every balanced diet before we go into meal planning. These are the vital nutrients that your body needs in big amounts to operate at its best. Carbohydrates, proteins, and fats are the three main macronutrients, and each has a specific function in your path toward nutrition and fitness.

Carbohydrates: Frequently regarded as the body's main source of energy, they provide the fuel required for regular activities and exercises. We'll talk about the distinction between complex and simple carbohydrates, how they affect blood sugar levels, and how to use them wisely in your meals.

Proteins are the foundation of muscle and are necessary for both tissue development and repair. Learn how to determine your protein needs depending on your fitness objectives and about sources that are not only tasty but also very protein-rich.

Contrary to common opinion, fats are an essential component of a healthy diet. We'll debunk the myths surrounding healthy fats, explain how they affect hormone production, and provide helpful advice for selecting the best fats for your meals.

Tips for Successful Meal Planning Adapted to Fitness Objectives

Meal planning is a deliberate method to obtain your intended fitness objectives; it goes beyond just preparing three balanced meals per day. Here are some helpful hints to get you going:

Set Specific Objectives: Decide if your fitness goals are to lose weight, build muscle, or enhance endurance. Your food plan will reflect your objectives.

Know Your Numbers: Recognize the ratios of your daily calorie requirements and macronutrients depending on your objectives. We'll simplify the procedure and walk you through the computations.

Learn about the advantages of taking regular, wholesome meals throughout the day and how they might enhance your metabolism in this section on meal frequency.

Explore the significance of eating a diverse diet to make sure you get a variety of nutrients. We'll demonstrate how to get the ideal balance.

Discover time-saving meal preparation techniques and the significance of portion management in controlling your calorie consumption.

How to Make a Customized Meal Plan for Your Needs

It's time to put theory into action and create a personalized food plan for you. We'll walk you through each stage of the procedure, assisting you to:

Choose your favorite dishes and tastes to make your meal plan fun and enduring.

Regardless of whether you're a busy professional or a serious athlete, modify your food plan to suit your lifestyle.

Make a weekly food plan that reflects your macronutrient and calorie objectives.

To simplify your food purchases and save waste, create a shopping list.

By the time you finish reading this chapter, you'll not only have a thorough grasp of macronutrients and how they fit into your diet but you'll also be prepared to start your unique meal-planning adventure. This chapter is your guide to making informed decisions in the kitchen, which can improve your body and health. So let's begin your journey to a stronger, leaner version of yourself.

Chapter 3

Recipe Categories

In our culinary quest to become a healthier, leaner, and stronger version of ourselves, Chapter 3 offers a fascinating introduction to the world of delectable and varied recipe categories created especially to support your fitness objectives. Here, we set out on a savory journey that will transform how you see food.

BREAKFAST ENHANCERS

1. Oatmeal Bowl Packed With Power

Start the day off right with a filling bowl of nutritious oatmeal that is naturally sweet.

Size of Serving: 1

Ten minutes for cooking and preparation

Ingredients:

- 1/2 cup rolled oats
- almond milk, 1 cup
- 1 banana, cut when ripe
- 1 teaspoon of honey
- 1/4 cup chopped nuts, such as walnuts or almonds

Instructions:

1. Oats should be added to boiling almond milk and simmered for 5 minutes.

2. Slices of banana, honey, and chopped almonds are added on top. Enjoy!

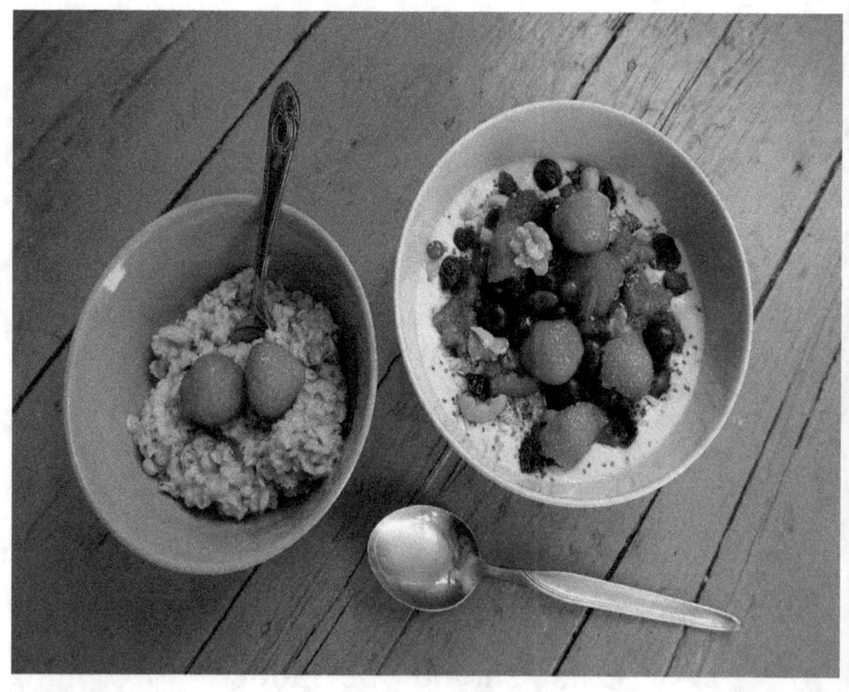

2. Scrambled Eggs Packed with Protein

Boost your morning energy with high-protein scrambled eggs.

Servings: 2

Ten minutes for cooking and preparation

Ingredients:

- Four big eggs
- chopped 1/4 cup spinach
- 14 cups of bell peppers, diced
- tomato dice, one-fourth cup
- pepper and salt as desired

Instructions:

1. Salt and pepper the eggs in a bowl after whisking them.
2. Vegetables are added to a hot nonstick pan and sautéed for 2 minutes.

3. Add eggs, scramble, and cook to your preferred doneness.

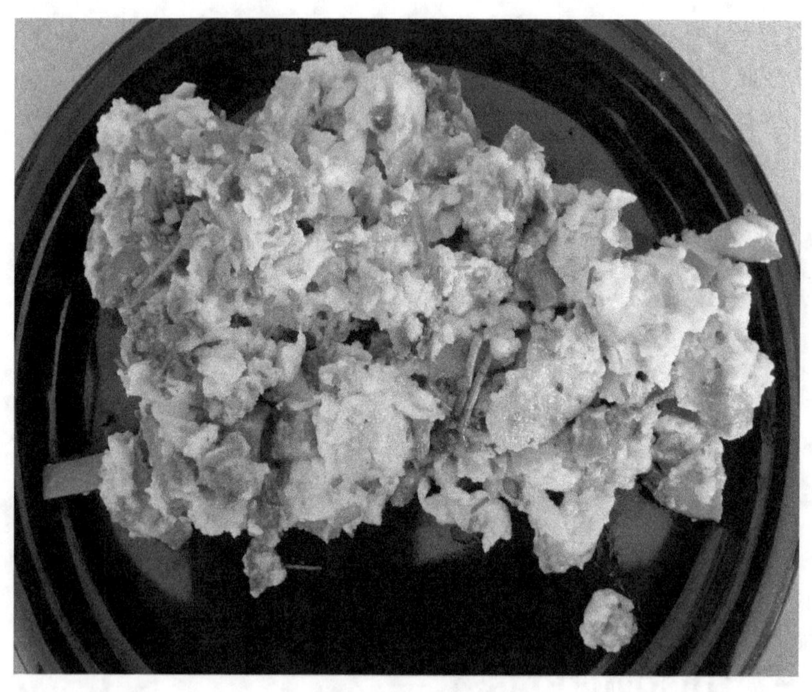

3. Invigorating Smoothie Bowl

In a nutshell: A hydrating and filling smoothie bowl to start your day.

Size of Serving: 1

Cooking and preparation time: 5 minutes

Ingredients:

- one banana, frozen
- Greek yogurt, half a cup
- Strawberries, blueberries, and raspberries totaling 1/2 cup
- 1 teaspoon of honey
- Granola, chia seeds, and fruit slices as toppings

Instructions:

1. Bananas, yogurt, mixed berries, and honey should all be well blended.
2. Pour into a bowl and top with fruit slices, granola, and chia seeds.

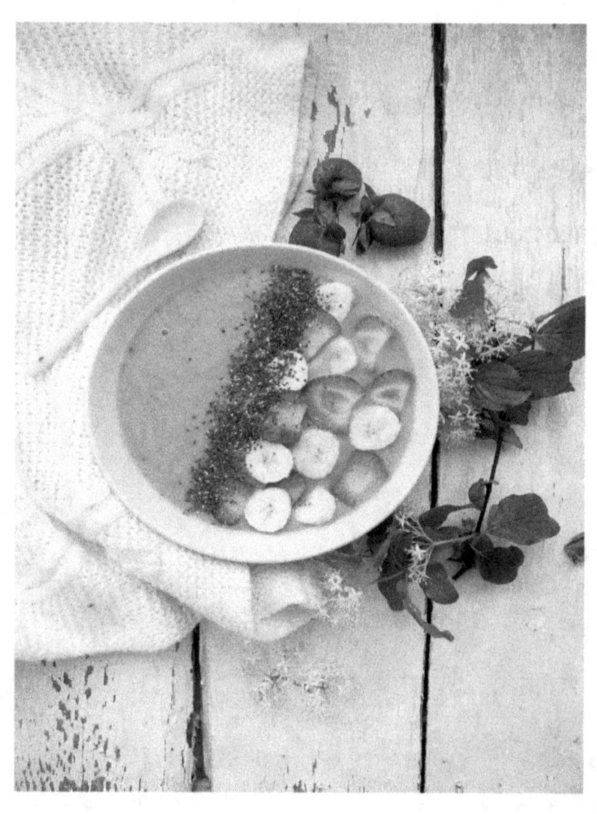

4. Breakfast Wrap with Avocado and Egg

A filling breakfast wrap including the delights of eggs and avocados.

Size of Serving: 1

15 minutes for cooking and preparation

Ingredients:

- 1 tortilla whole-wheat
- 1 mashed, ripe avocado
- 2 scrambled eggs
- Optional salsa or spicy sauce

Instructions:

1. In a pan or the microwave, reheat the tortilla.
2. Spread the tortilla with mashed avocado.
3. Add salsa and scrambled eggs, if preferred.

4. Take a seat and enjoy!

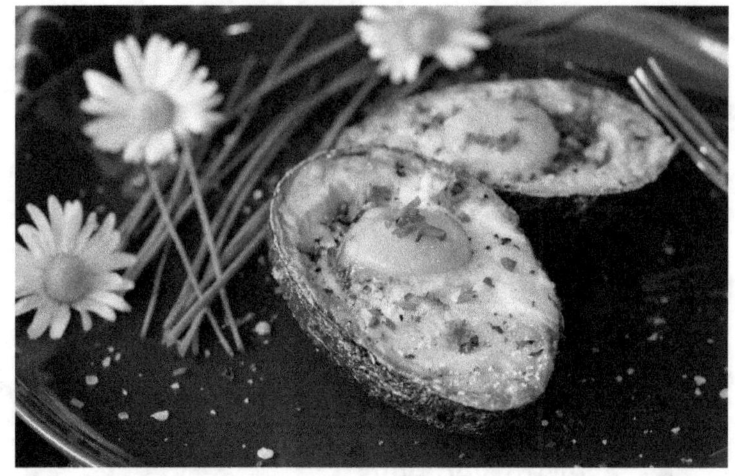

5. Smoothie with Peanut Butter and Bananas

A smoothie that is creamy and protein-rich and has a traditional taste combination.

Size of Serving: 1

Cooking and preparation time: 5 minutes

Ingredients:

- one ripe banana
- 2/fourths cup peanut butter
- Almond milk, 1 cup
- 1 tablespoon of optional honey
- An ice cube

Instructions:

1. Smoothly combine banana, peanut butter, almond milk, honey (if using), and ice cubes.

2. These dishes provide you with many alternatives for filling your mornings

with wholesome and delectable breakfast options.

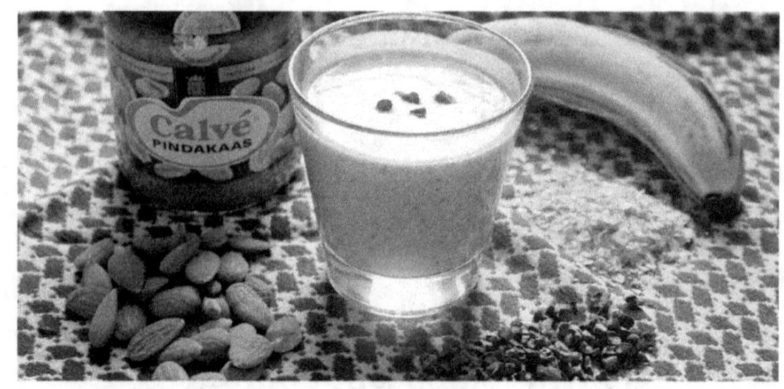

6. Oats Berry Bliss Overnight

A no-cook, make-ahead breakfast packed with berries that are high in antioxidants.

Size of Serving: 1

5 minutes for preparation and cooking (plus chilling for the night).

Ingredients:

- 1/2 cup rolled oats
- Greek yogurt, half a cup
- Berry mixture of blueberries, raspberries, and strawberries, 1/2 cup
- 1 teaspoon of honey

Instructions:

1. Oats, Greek yogurt, fruit, and honey should be arranged in a container.
2. Overnight, cover and chill. Before enjoying, stir.

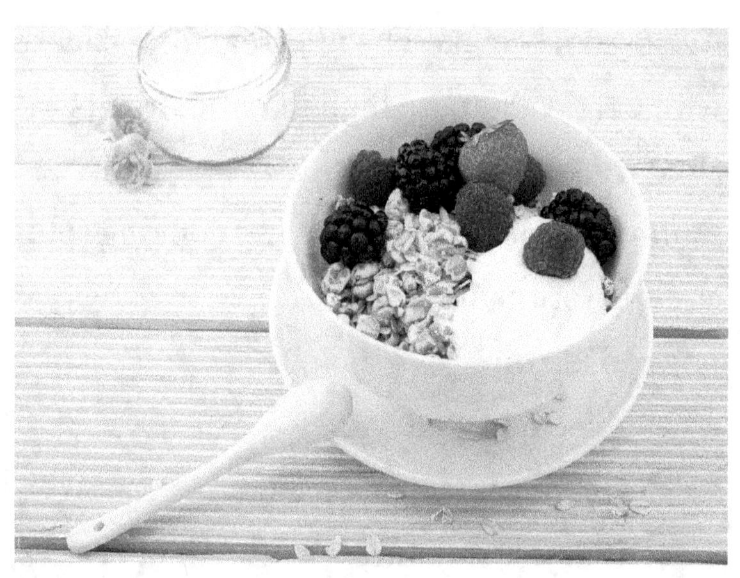

7. Breakfast Burrito Packed With Veggies

A filling breakfast burrito loaded with vibrant veggies.

Size of Serving: 1

15 minutes for cooking and preparation

Ingredients:

- 1 tortilla whole-wheat
- 2 scrambled eggs
- 14 cups of bell peppers, diced
- onions, diced, 14 cup
- tomato dice, one-fourth cup
- Optional salsa or spicy sauce

Instructions:

1. Scrambled eggs, bell peppers, onions, and tomatoes should all be placed within the tortilla.

2. For more taste, mix with salsa or spicy
    sauce.

3. Enjoy by folding it into a tortilla!

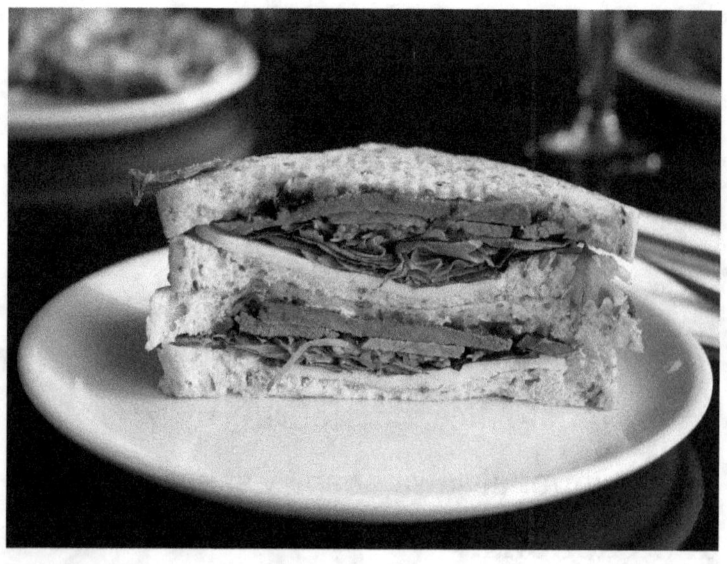

8. Green Goddess Smoothie

A green smoothie that is colorful and nutrient-rich.

Size of Serving: 1

Cooking and preparation time: 5 minutes

Ingredients:

- spinach leaves, 1 cup
- Ripe banana, half
- 1/2 cup pieces of pineapple
- Unsweetened coconut milk in a half-cup
- Chia seeds, one tablespoon

Instructions:

Smoothly combine spinach, banana, pineapple, coconut milk, and chia seeds.

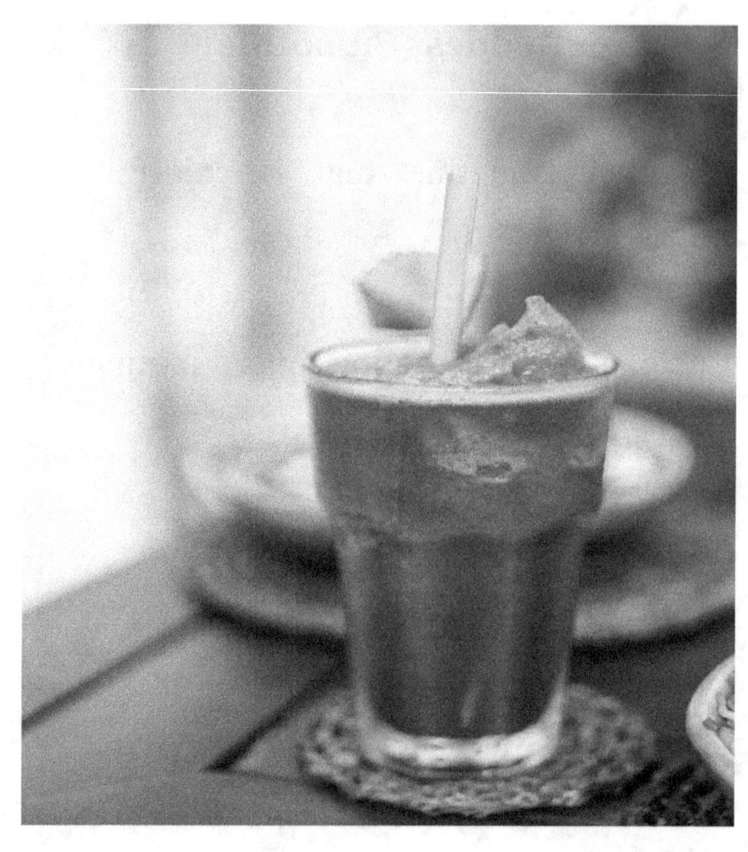

9. Breakfast Bowl with Quinoa

A breakfast dish high in protein that includes quinoa and fresh fruit.

Size of Serving: 1

20 minutes are spent cooking and preparing.

Ingredients:

- half a cup of cooked quinoa
- Greek yogurt, half a cup
- 1/2 cup of assorted fruits, such as berries, mango, and kiwis
- 1 teaspoon of honey
- chopped nuts, if desired

Instructions:

Quinoa, Greek yogurt, mixed fruits, honey, and chopped nuts (if preferred) should be arranged in a bowl.

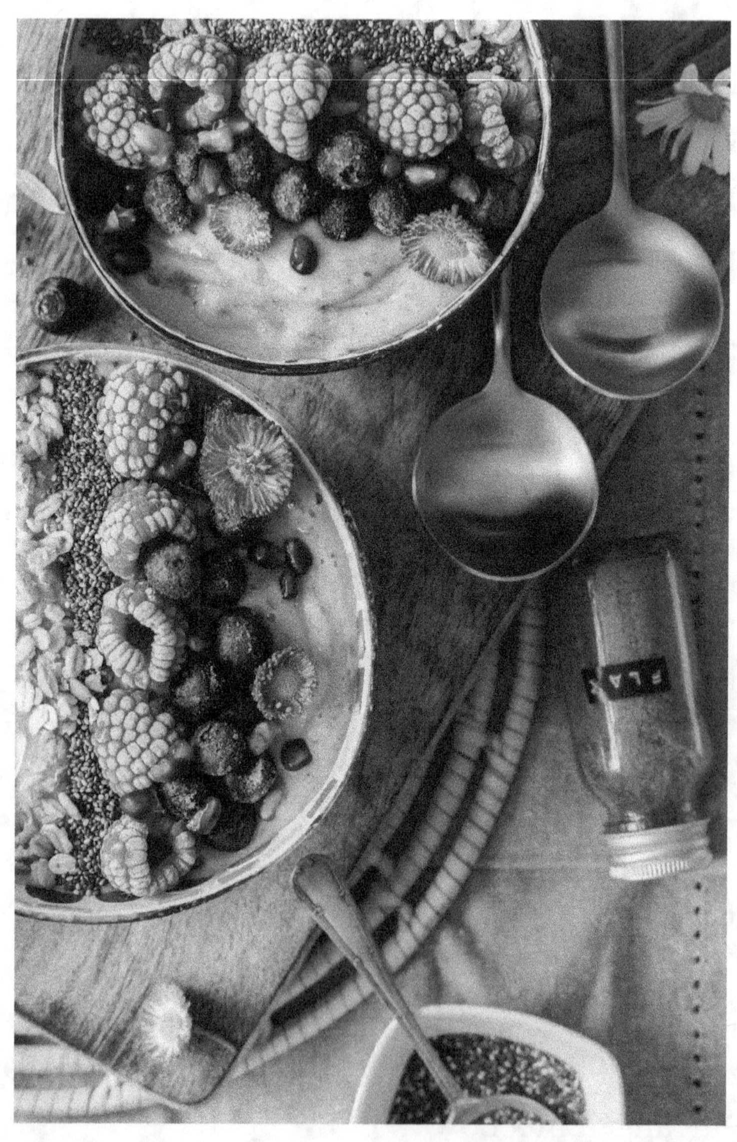

10. Parfait with chia seed pudding

A chia seed pudding parfait with layers of taste that is healthy.

Serving size is one.

10 minutes for preparation and cooking (plus chilling time)

- Substances:
- Chia seeds, 2 teaspoons
- One cup of almond milk
- 1/2 cup mangos, diced
- 14 cups of granola
- Optional: 1 tablespoon maple syrup

Requirements:

1. Mix almond milk with chia seeds. It will thicken after a few hours or an overnight rest in the refrigerator.

2. Chia pudding, sliced mango, granola, and maple syrup (if preferred) should be layered in a glass.

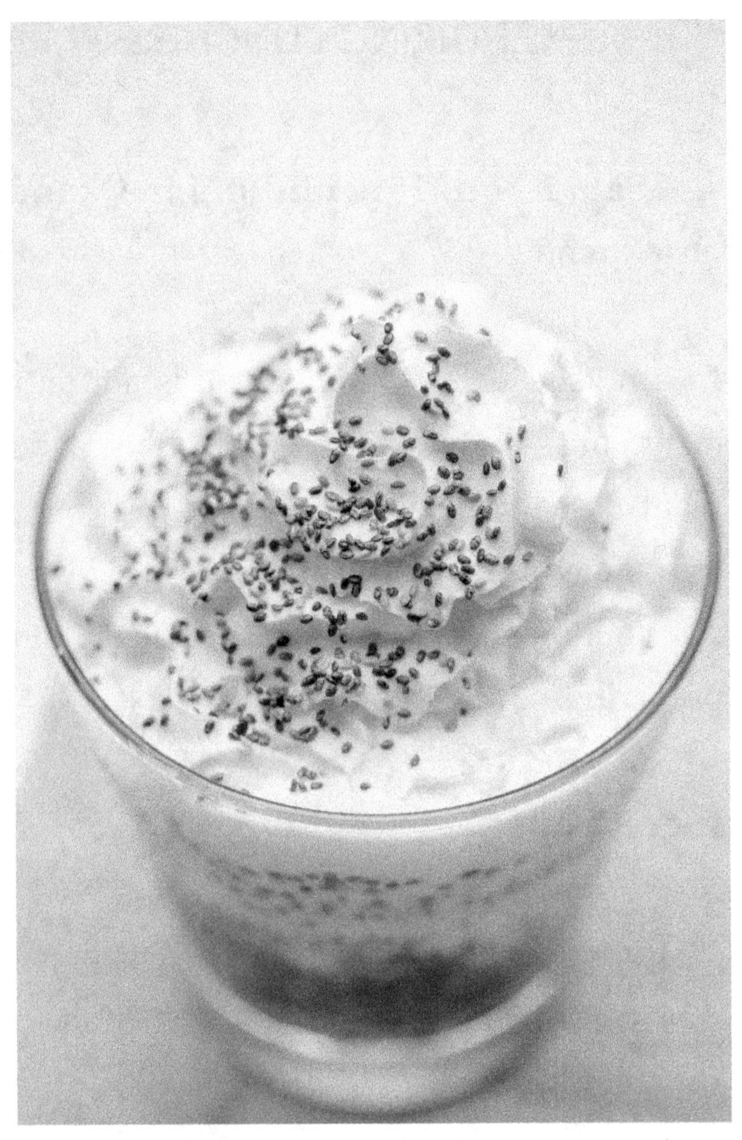

1. Salad bowl with quinoa and chickpeas

In a nutshell, this vibrant salad is not only tasty but also loaded with fiber and plant-based protein.

Two servings per recipe

20 minutes are spent cooking and preparing.

Ingredients:

- cooked quinoa, 1 cup
- 1 can (15 oz) washed and drained chickpeas
- 1 cup halved cherry tomatoes

- cuke, one, diced
- 14 cup coarsely chopped red onion
- 14 cup chopped fresh parsley
- Olive oil, two teaspoons
- lemon juice from one
- pepper and salt as desired

Instructions:

1. Quinoa, chickpeas, cherry tomatoes, cucumber, red onion, and parsley should all be combined in a big dish.
2. Mix the olive oil, lemon juice, salt, and pepper in a separate small bowl.
3. After adding the dressing, toss the salad to get a uniform coating.
4. Either serve right now or store in the fridge.

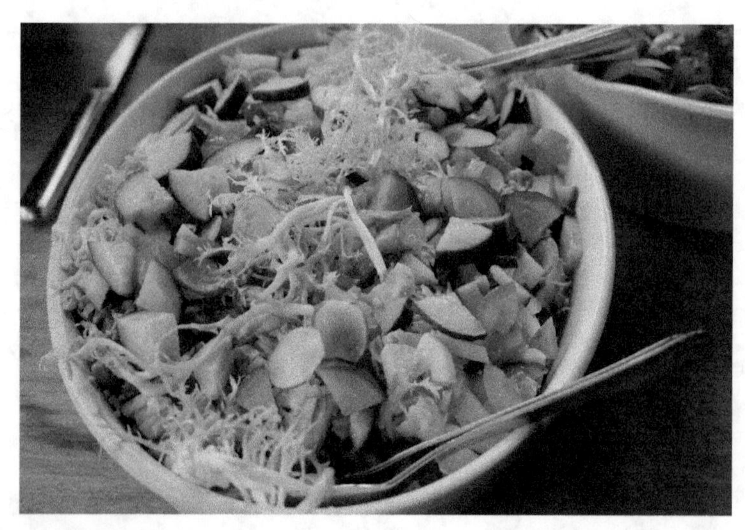

2. Wrap with avocado and turkey

A wrap that is high in protein and made with lean turkey and smooth avocado.

Size of Serving: 1 wrap

Ten minutes for cooking and preparation

Ingredients:

- 1 tortilla whole-wheat
- 4 turkey breast slices
- sliced avocado, half
- 4 cups of spinach leaves
- 1/fourth cup Greek yogurt
- Dijon mustard, 1 teaspoon

Instructions:

1. The whole-wheat tortilla should be laid flat.
2. The tortilla should be covered with Greek yogurt and Dijon mustard.

3. Layer spinach leaves, avocado slices, and turkey slices.

4. Slice the tortilla in half after securely rolling it up.

3. Bell Peppers Stuffed with Spinach and Quinoa

These stuffed bell peppers make for a full and healthy lunch alternative.

Size of Serving: Two stuffed peppers

Cooking and preparation time: 45 minutes

Ingredients:

- two any-color bell peppers, two
- cooked quinoa, 1 cup

- 1 cup chopped fresh spinach
- 1/2 cup washed and drained black beans
- a half-cup of corn kernels
- tomato dice, half a cup
- 1/8 tsp. cumin
- pepper and salt as desired
- (Optional) 1/4 cup shredded cheddar cheese

Instructions:

1. Set the oven's temperature to 375°F (190°C).
2. Bell peppers need to have their tops removed and their seeds removed.
3. Quinoa, chopped spinach, black beans, corn, diced tomatoes, cumin, salt, and pepper should all be combined in a big dish.

4. Stuff the quinoa mixture inside each bell pepper.

5. Bake the filled peppers for 30-35 minutes on a baking dish with foil covering them.

6. Remove the foil, top with cheese, and bake for an additional 5 minutes, or until the cheese is melted and bubbling, if preferred.

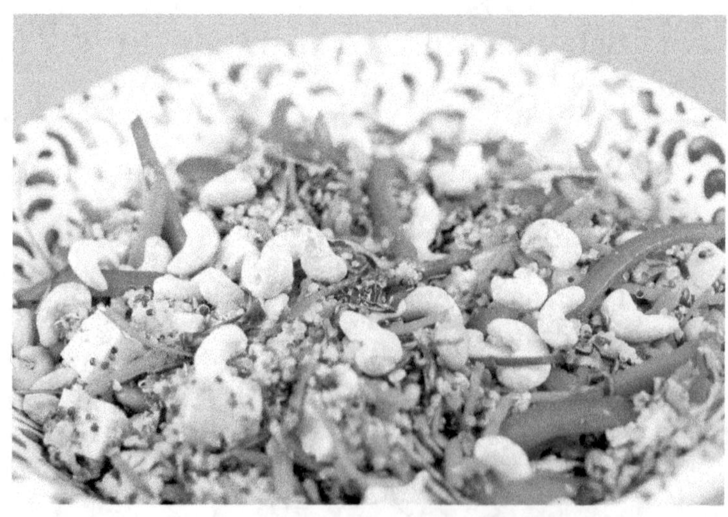

4. Stir-fry with Chicken and Veggies

An efficient and filling stir-fry that's ideal for a lunchtime energy boost.

Two servings per recipe

Cooking and preparation time: 25 minutes

Ingredients:

- 2 cubed, skinless, boneless chicken breasts
- broccoli florets in a cup
- 1 finely sliced bell pepper
- 1 finely sliced carrot
- 2 minced garlic cloves
- Low-sodium soy sauce, two teaspoons
- 1 teaspoon of honey
- 1 teaspoon grated ginger

- Vegetable oil, 1 tablespoon
- brown rice prepared for serving

Instructions:

1. Combine soy sauce, honey, and grated ginger in a small bowl.
2. Using a large pan over medium-high heat, warm the vegetable oil.
3. Add the chicken cubes and simmer for 5 to 7 minutes, or until well browned. Take out of the skillet.
4. Garlic, broccoli, bell pepper, and carrot may all be added to the same pan. The vegetables should be tender-crisp after 3–4 minutes of stirring.
5. Add the sauce to the pan with the cooked chicken back in it. Stir-fry for a further two to three minutes.

6. the stir-fry over brown rice that has been prepared.

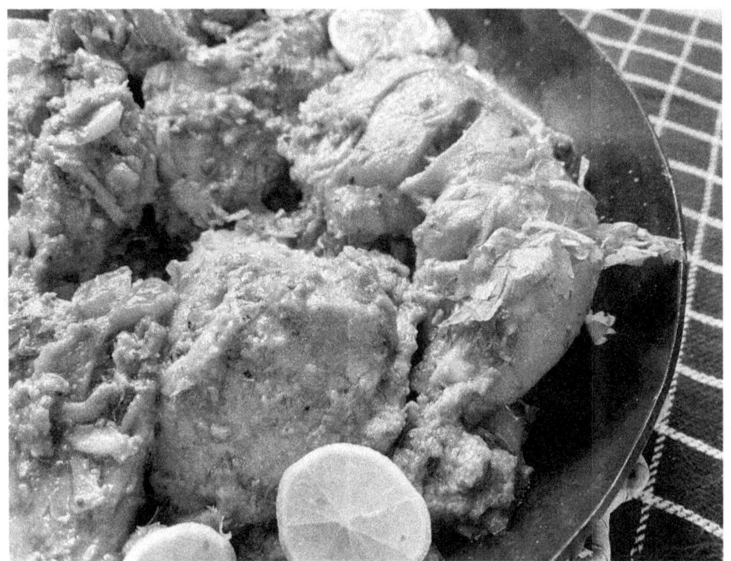

5. White bean and tuna salad

Using tuna, white beans, and fresh veggies, this salad is protein-rich.

Two servings per recipe

15 minutes for cooking and preparation

Ingredients:

- 2 cans of tuna in water, each 5 ounces, drained
- 1 can (15 oz) washed and drained white beans
- 1/2 red onion, chopped finely
- Half a cup of cherry tomatoes
- Pitted and sliced Kalamata olives, 1/4 cup
- Olive oil, two teaspoons
- lemon juice from one
- pepper and salt as desired

Instructions:

1. Tuna, white beans, red onion, cherry tomatoes, and Kalamata olives should all be combined in a big dish.

2. Lemon juice and olive oil should be drizzled over. Add salt and pepper to taste.

3. Serve after tossing to mix.

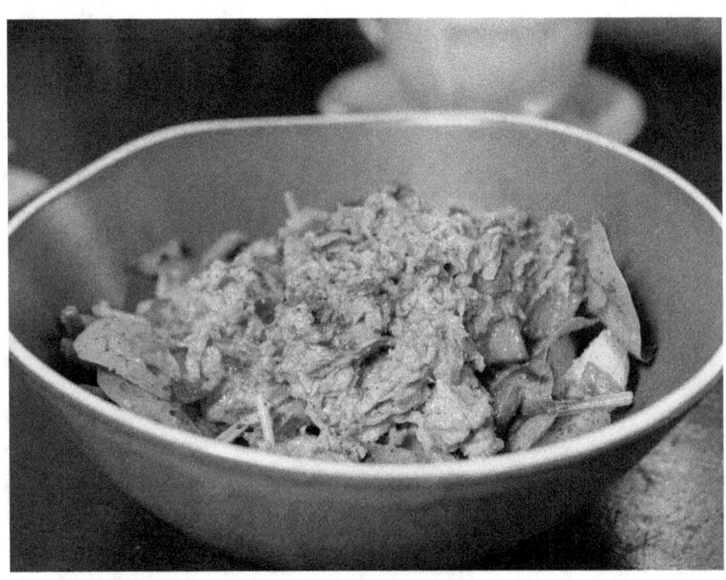

6. Burrito Bowl with Sweet Potato and Black Beans

Roasted sweet potatoes, black beans, and tasty garnishes make up this burrito bowl.

Two servings per recipe

30-minute preparation and cooking time

Ingredients:

- 2 cups of brown rice, cooked
- 2 tiny sweet potatoes, diced after being peeled
- 1 can (15 oz) washed and drained black beans
- 1 cup fresh or frozen corn kernels
- 1 sliced avocado
- chopped 1/4 cup cilantro
- 1/4 cup of unsweetened Greek yogurt
- wedges sliced from 1 lime

- (Optional) Hot sauce

Instructions:

1. Set the oven's temperature to 400°F (200°C). Olive oil should be drizzled over the sweet potato cubes before roasting for **20 to 25 minutes**, or until they are soft but still somewhat crunchy.

2. two bowls of brown rice that have been prepared.

3. Add roasted sweet potatoes, black beans, corn, pieces of avocado, and cilantro to the top.

4. Pour Greek yogurt over the dish and top with slices of lime.

5. If you want, add spicy sauce.

7.   Quinoa   Salad   from   the Mediterranean

A salad with Mediterranean characteristics that is protein-rich and refreshing.

Two servings per recipe

20 minutes are spent cooking and preparing.

Ingredients:

- cooked quinoa, 1 cup
- sliced cucumber, half a cup
- Half a cup of cherry tomatoes
- 14 cup coarsely chopped red onion
- Pitted and sliced Kalamata olives, 1/4 cup
- 2 teaspoons of crumbled feta cheese
- 2 teaspoons chopped fresh basil
- Olive oil, two teaspoons

- lemon juice from one
- pepper and salt as desired

Instructions:

1. Quinoa, cucumber, cherry tomatoes, red onion, Kalamata olives, feta cheese, and fresh basil should all be combined in a big dish.
2. Lemon juice and olive oil should be drizzled over. Add salt and pepper to taste.
3. Serve after tossing to mix.

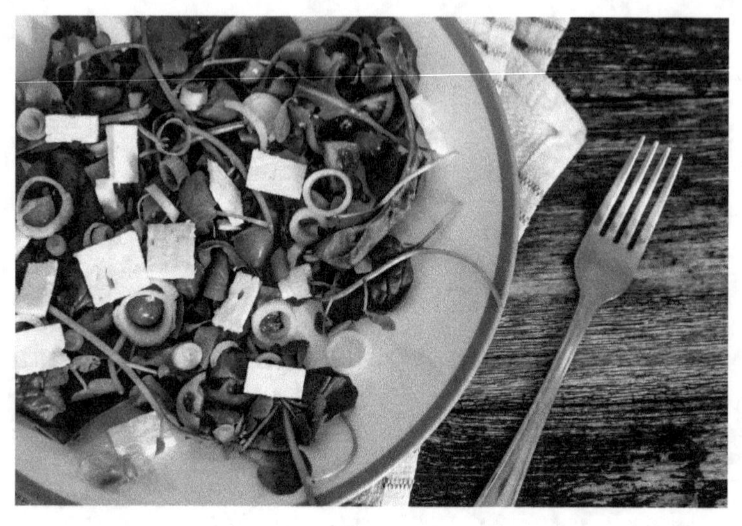

8. Soup with Lentils and Veggies

A filling and healthy soup packed with colorful veggies and lentils.

4 servings per item.

Cooking and preparation time: 45 minutes

Ingredients:

- 1 cup washed dry green or brown lentils
- one sliced onion
- 2 sliced carrots
- 2 diced celery stalks
- 2 minced garlic cloves
- 1 can of chopped tomatoes (14 oz).
- Six cups of vegetable stock
- 1/9 cup cumin
- smoked paprika, 1 teaspoon

- pepper and salt as desired
- garnishing with fresh parsley

Instructions:

1. Olive oil is heated over medium heat in a big saucepan. Add the celery, onion, carrots, and garlic. Sauté until softened for 5 to 7 minutes.
2. Add the lentils, tomatoes, cumin, smoked paprika, salt, and pepper along with the vegetable broth.
3. When the lentils are ready, simmer for 30-35 minutes after bringing them to a boil.
4. Serve hot with fresh parsley as a garnish.

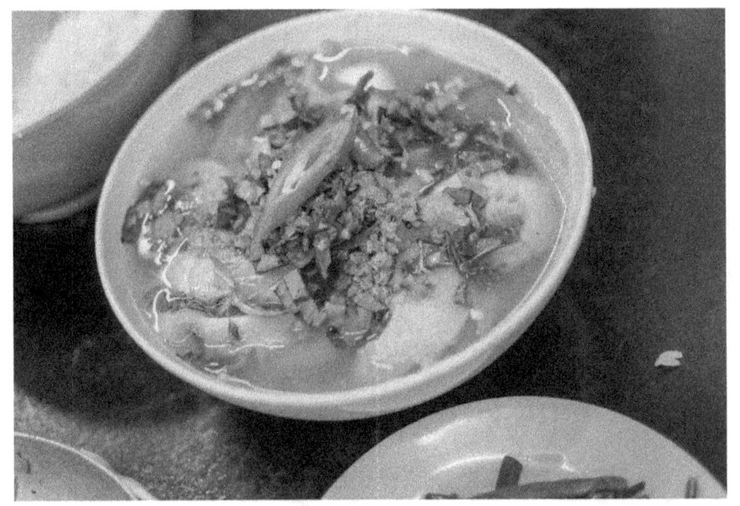

9. Chinese-style chicken salad

An Asian-inspired salad that is tasty and high in protein.

Two servings per recipe

Cooking and preparation time: 25 minutes

Ingredients:
- 2 skinless, boneless breasts of chicken
- 4 cups mixed greens, such as romaine, spinach, and arugula
- 1 cup of purple cabbage, chopped
- a cup of grated carrots
- Peanuts, chopped, 14 cup
- Sesame seeds, 2 teaspoons
- 2 chopped green onions
- A quarter cup of Asian salad dressing

Instructions:

1. Chicken breasts should be salted and peppered. Cook thoroughly on the grill or in a pan for 6 to 8 minutes each side. Cut into long, thin strips.
2. Combine mixed greens, shredded carrots, shredded cabbage, chopped peanuts, sesame seeds, and finely chopped green onions in a big bowl.
3. Add cooked chicken slices on top.
4. Add an Asian salad dressing and blend by drizzling it over the salad.

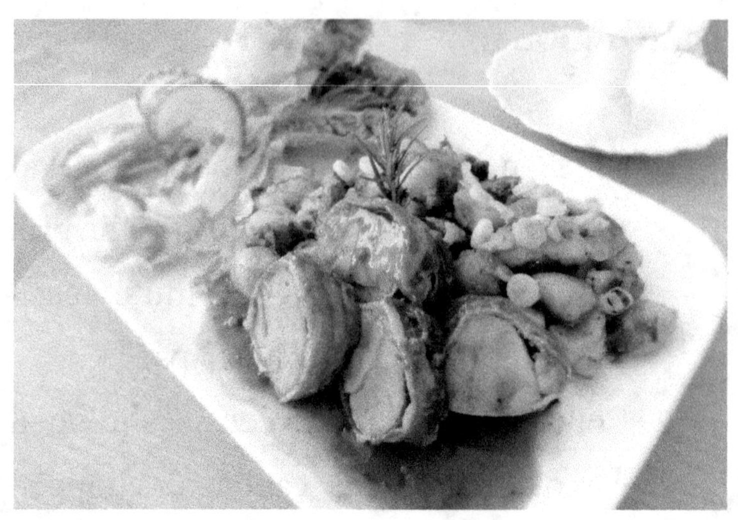

10. Hummus and Veggie Wrap

A simple and filling vegetable wrap with smooth hummus.

Size of Serving: 1 wrap

Ten minutes for cooking and preparation

Ingredients:

- 1 tortilla whole-wheat
- two teaspoons of hummus
- baby spinach leaves, half a cup
- 14 cups of cucumber slices
- Sliced bell pepper, 1/4 cup
- Carrots, shredded, 14 cup
- Alfalfa sprouts, 1/4 cup (optional)
- pepper and salt as desired

Instructions:

1. The whole-wheat tortilla should be laid flat.
2. On the tortilla, equally, distribute the hummus.
3. Baby spinach leaves, diced bell pepper, diced cucumber, shredded carrots, and alfalfa sprouts (if used) should be arranged in layers.
4. Add salt and pepper to taste.
5. Slice the tortilla in half after securely rolling it up.

These nutrient-rich lunch meals are packed with taste and appeal to a target market that values good health and physical fitness. Enjoy your delicious and filling meals!

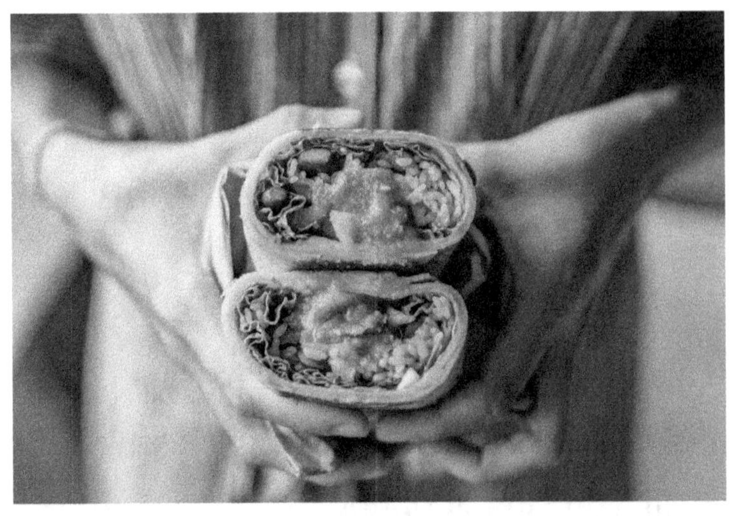

1. Chicken with Grilled Lemon and Herbs

This tangy grilled chicken is marinated in a tasty lemon herb combination, making it the ideal light supper option.

4 servings per item.

Time to Prepare & Cook: 30 minutes

Ingredients:

- 4 skinless, boneless breasts of chicken
- zest and juice from two lemons
- 2 minced garlic cloves
- 2 teaspoons chopped fresh rosemary
- Olive oil, two teaspoons
- pepper and salt as desired

Instructions:

1. Lemon juice, zest, garlic, rosemary, olive oil, salt, and pepper should all be combined in a bowl.

2. For 20 minutes, marinate the chicken in the mixture.

3. Cook the chicken on the grill over medium-high heat for 6–7 minutes on each side.

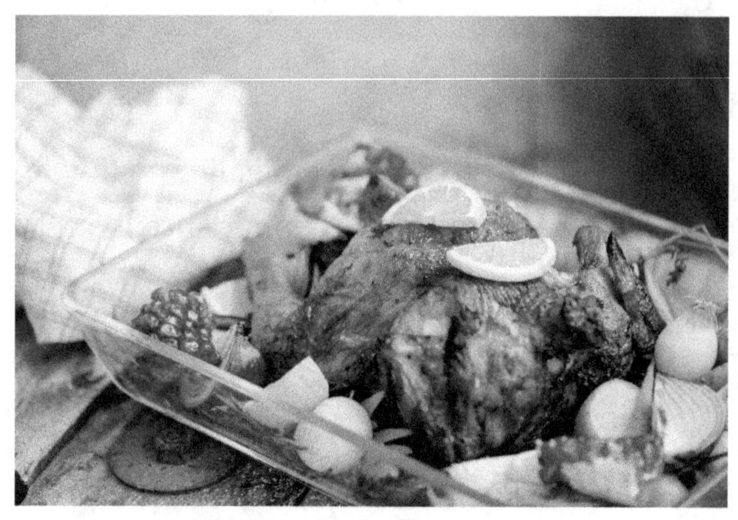

2. Aglio e Olio spaghetti

A traditional Italian meal made with three tasty yet straightforward ingredients: garlic, olive oil, and red pepper flakes.

Two servings per recipe

Time to Prepare & Cook: 15 minutes

Ingredients:

- 80 g of pasta
- 4 finely sliced garlic cloves
- Olive oil, 1/4 cup
- Red pepper flakes in the amount of half
- chopped fresh parsley for a garnish
- Parmesan cheese, grated (optional)

Instructions:

1. Follow the directions on the spaghetti's packaging for cooking.

2. Olive oil should be heated in a skillet before adding the garlic and red pepper flakes.

3. Cooked spaghetti is combined with the garlic and oil.

4. If preferred, add fresh parsley and Parmesan cheese as a garnish.

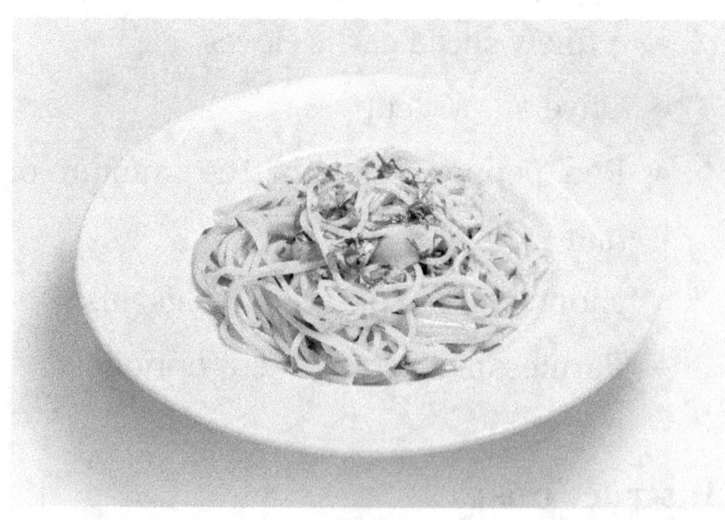

3. Salmon with Balsamic Glaze

Salmon filets with a sweet and tart balsamic glaze go well beautifully.

Two servings per recipe

20 minutes for preparation and cooking

Ingredients:

- 2 filets of salmon
- Balsamic vinegar, 1/4 cup
- Honey, two tablespoons
- 1 minced garlic clove
- pepper and salt as desired

Instructions:

Set the oven's temperature to 375°F (190°C).

1. Balsamic vinegar, honey, garlic, salt, and pepper are combined in a small pot. until it thickens, simmer.

2. The glaze should be applied to the salmon filets before baking for 15 minutes or until done.

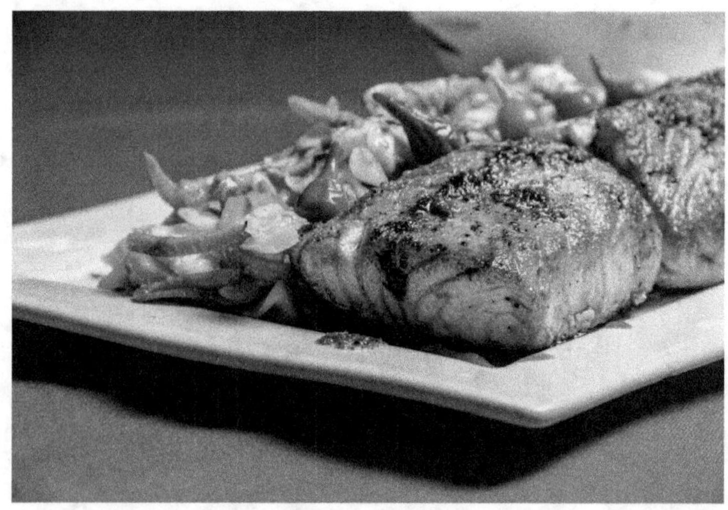

4. Thai Green Curry for Vegetarians

A delicious and fragrant Thai green curry packed with vibrant veggies and tofu.

4 servings per item.

25 minutes for preparation and cooking

Ingredients:

- 1 cubed block of tofu
- 2 cups of mixed veggies, including carrots, bell peppers, and zucchini
- Green curry paste, two teaspoons
- One 14-ounce can of coconut milk
- a serving of soy sauce
- For garnish, use fresh basil leaves

Instructions:

1. Sauté tofu in a pan until it becomes golden. Take out and put aside.

2. Add curry paste to the same pan and
   cook for a minute.

3. five minutes after adding the mixed
   veggies.

4. Add soy sauce and coconut milk and
   stir. Simmer the veggies until they are
   ready.

5. Re-add the tofu to the pan and reheat.

6. Serve over rice or noodles with fresh
   basil leaves.

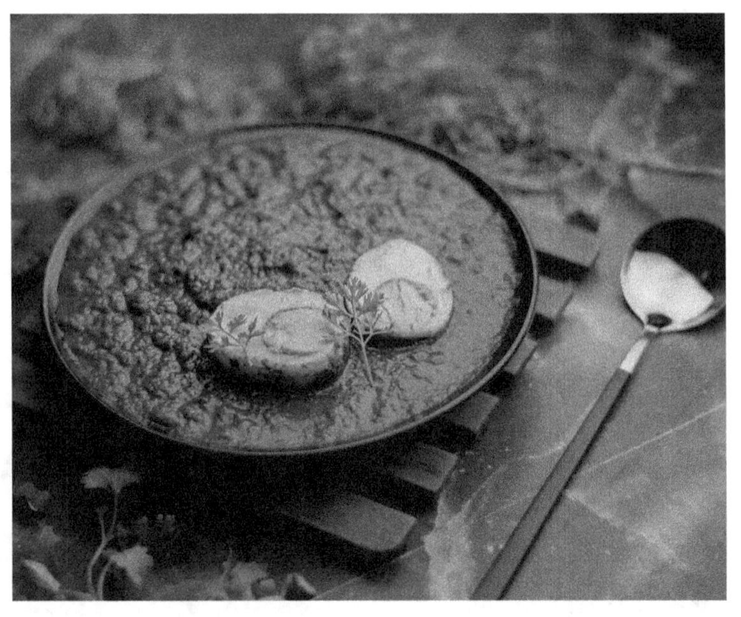

5. Bell Peppers Stuffed with Quinoa

Bright bell peppers stuffed with a filling made of quinoa and vegetables.

4 servings per item.

45 minutes for preparation and cooking

Ingredients:

- 4 big bell peppers, seeded and cut in half.
- 1 cup cooked quinoa
- 1 cup cooked black beans
- Corn kernels, 1 cup
- Diced tomatoes, 1 cup
- (Optional) 1/2 cup shredded cheese
- 1/9 cup cumin
- pepper and salt as desired

Instructions:

1. Set the oven's temperature to 375°F (190°C).

2. Cooked quinoa, black beans, corn, chopped tomatoes, cumin, salt, and pepper should all be combined in a dish.

3. The quinoa mixture should be placed into each bell pepper half.

4. If you want, add some cheese shredded on top.

5. Bake peppers for 25 to 30 minutes, or until they are soft.

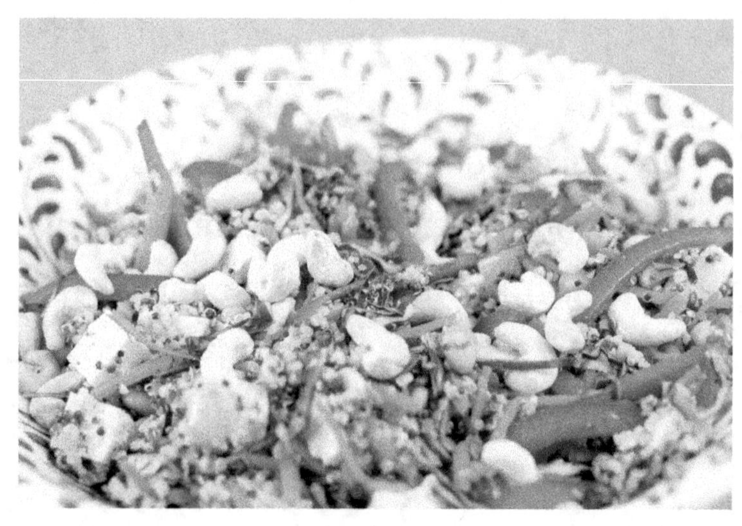

6. Chickpea Salad from the Mediterranean

A light and healthy salad made with chickpeas, tomatoes, cucumbers, and other Mediterranean ingredients.

4 servings per item.

Time to Prepare & Cook: 15 minutes

Ingredients:

- 2 cans of chickpeas (15 oz each), drained and rinsed

cuke, one, diced

- 2 cups halved cherry tomatoes
- 1/2 cup coarsely chopped red onion
- 14 cup chopped fresh parsley
- Crumbled 1/4 cup feta cheese, if desired

- 3 tablespoons of olive oil, 2 teaspoons of lemon juice, 1 chopped garlic clove, salt, and pepper make up the dressing.

Instructions:

1. Chickpeas, cucumber, cherry tomatoes, red onion, and parsley should all be combined in a big bowl.
2. Mix the ingredients for the dressing in a small dish.
3. Over the salad, drizzle the dressing, and mix to blend.
4. If desired, add some crumbled feta cheese on top.

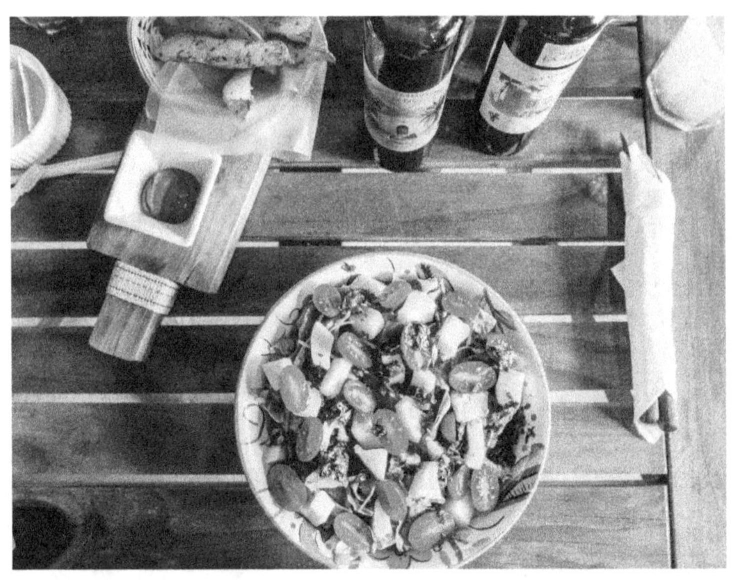

7. Broccoli and Snow Pea Stir-Fry with Beef

Quick and delectable stir-fry of beef with veggies that are crisp and a tasty sauce.

4 servings per item.

20 minutes for preparation and cooking

Ingredients:

- 1 pound of finely cut flank steak
- 200 grams of broccoli florets
- 1 cup trimmed snow peas
- 1 sliced red bell pepper
- 3 minced garlic cloves
- 2/fourths cup soy sauce
- 1/fourth cup of oyster sauce
- Sesame oil, 1 teaspoon
- Vegetable oil, two teaspoons

Instructions:

1. Vegetable oil should be heated very quickly in a big pan or wok.

2. Stir-fry the beef slices for two to three minutes, or until browned. Take out of the skillet.

3. Garlic should be added to the same pan and stir-fried for 30 seconds.

4. Add bell pepper, broccoli, and snow peas. Vegetables should be stir-fried for 3–4 minutes or until crisp-tender.

5. Add soy sauce, oyster sauce, and sesame oil to the pan with the meat once more. For a further 2 minutes, stir-fry.

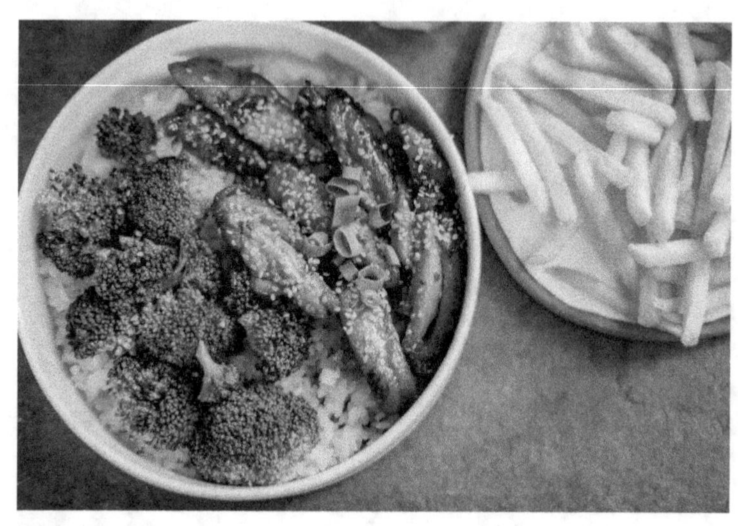

8. Portobello Stuffed Mushrooms

Portobello mushrooms stuffed with a flavorful blend of cheese, breadcrumbs, and spinach.

Two servings per recipe

25 minutes for preparation and cooking

Ingredients:

- Portobello mushrooms, four, big
- 2 cups chopped spinach
- a half-cup of breadcrumbs
- Shredded mozzarella cheese in a cup
- 2 minced garlic cloves
- Olive oil, two teaspoons
- pepper and salt as desired

Instructions:

1. Set the oven's temperature to 375°F (190°C).

2. The mushrooms' stems should be cut off, and the gills should be removed.

3. Garlic and spinach are sautéed in hot olive oil until the spinach wilts.

4. Sauteed spinach, breadcrumbs, mozzarella cheese, salt, and pepper should all be combined in a bowl.

5. Place the stuffed mushrooms on a baking sheet after stuffing each one.

6. Bake the topping until golden brown and the mushrooms are cooked through, about 15 to 20 minutes.

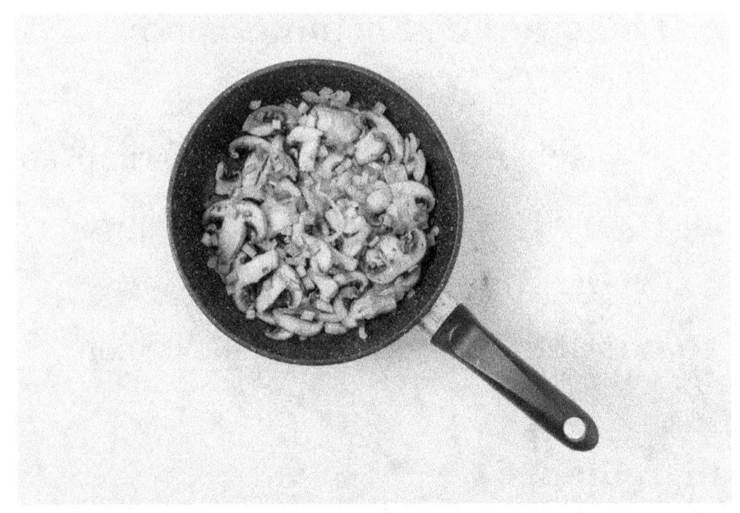

9. Linguine and Shrimp Scampi

Over linguine pasta, delectable shrimp are mixed in butter, garlic, and lemon sauce.
4 servings per item.
20 minutes for preparation and cooking

Ingredients:
- 8 ounces of linguine
- 1 pound of peeled and deveined big shrimp
- 4 minced garlic cloves
- White wine, 1/4 cup (optional)
- 1/fourth cup chicken broth
- lemon juice from one
- 2 teaspoons chopped fresh parsley
- Butter, two tablespoons
- pepper and salt as desired

Instructions:

1. Linguine should be prepared as directed on the packaging.
2. Melt butter in a pan and cook garlic until fragrant.
3. When the shrimp is pink on all sides, add them and simmer for 2-3 minutes.
4. Take the shrimp out of the pan.
5. White wine (if needed) should be used to deglaze the pan before chicken broth and lemon juice are added. For a few minutes, simmer.
6. Toss the cooked linguine in the sauce and return the shrimp to the pan.
7. Add salt and pepper to taste and garnish with fresh parsley.

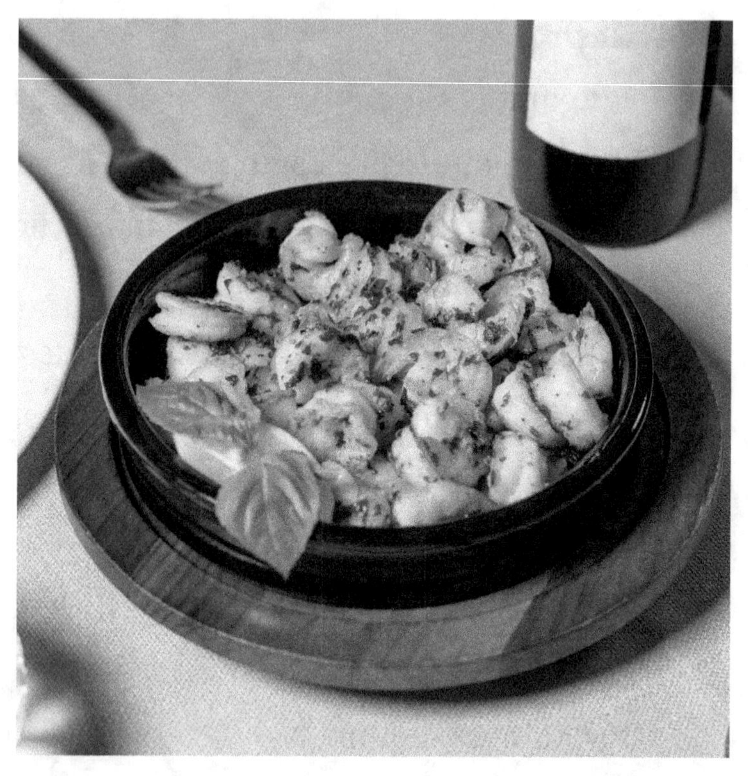

10. Vegan Chickpea and Sweet Potato Curry

Sweet potatoes and chickpeas are the main ingredients in this substantial and tasty vegan curry, which is served with a fragrant coconut milk sauce.

Servings Per Recipe: 4

30-minute prep and cooking time

Substances:

- 2 sweet potatoes, diced after being peeled
- 1 can (15 oz) washed and drained chickpeas
- One 14-ounce can of chopped tomatoes
- One 14-ounce can of coconut milk
- 1 finely chopped onion

- 2 minced garlic cloves
- Curry powder, 2 teaspoons
- One tablespoon cumin
- To taste, salt and pepper
- Fresh cilantro, for adornment

Requirements:

1. Garlic and onion should be cooked till transparent in a big saucepan.
2. Diced tomatoes, coconut milk, sweet potatoes, chickpeas, curry powder, and cumin are all good additions.
3. Cook sweet potatoes in a 20 to 25-minute simmer.
4. Add salt and pepper to taste.
5. Serve with fresh cilantro as a garnish over rice.

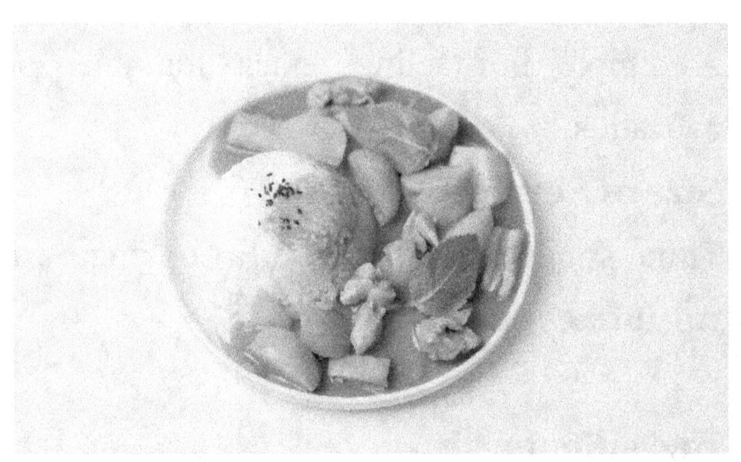

SNACKS RECIPES

1. Bites of avocado toast

A simple but filling snack for fans of avocados.

Size of Serving: 2 toasts

Time for Preparation and Cooking: **10 minutes**

Ingredients:

- Bread, two slices of whole grain
- 1 mature avocado
- halved cherry tomatoes
- pepper and salt as desired

Instructions:

1. Slices of whole-grain bread are toasted.

2. Spread the ripe avocado equally on the toast by mashing it.

3. Cherry tomatoes should be halved and salt and pepper should be added on top.

4. Serve each toast by slicing it into bite-sized pieces.

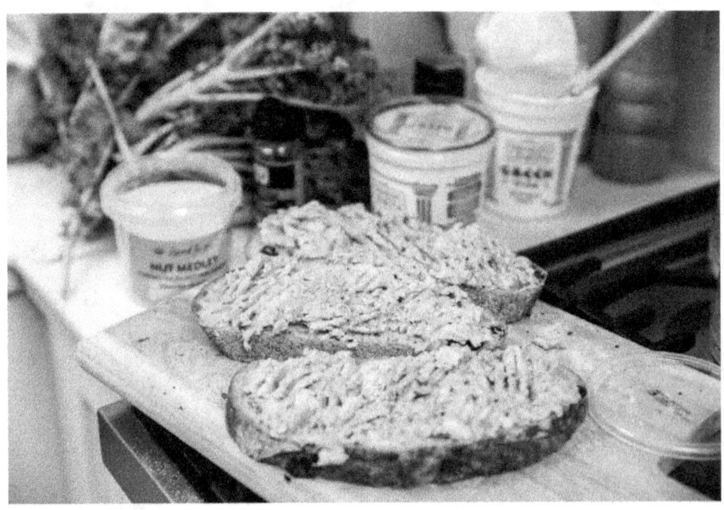

2. Parfait of Greek yogurt

A snack with a protein boost and a taste explosion.

Size of Serving: 1 parfait

Time for Preparation and Cooking: **5 minutes**

Ingredients:

- Greek yogurt, one cup
- 1/4 cup of cereal
- 1/4 cup of mixed berries, such as blueberries and strawberries
- For drizzling, use honey or maple syrup

Instructions:

1. Greek yogurt, granola, and mixed berries should be arranged in a glass or dish.

2. The layers should be repeated until the glass or bowl is full.

3. On top, drizzle some honey or maple syrup.

4. Relax for a while, then have pleasure!

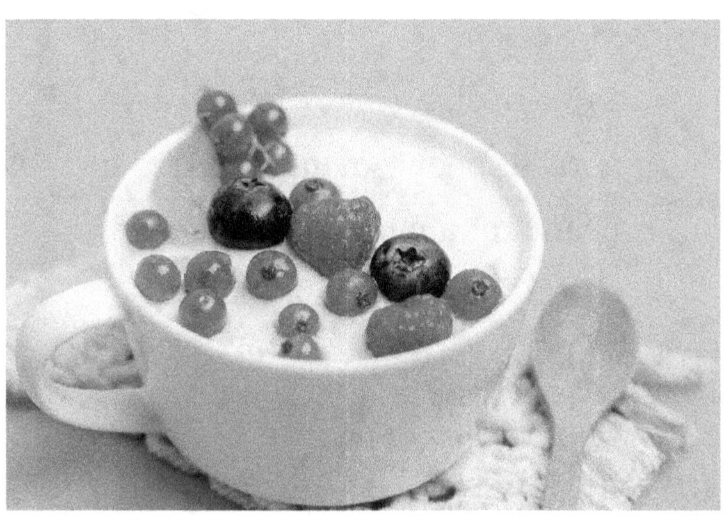

3. Banana and Nut Butter Rice Cakes

Described as a combination of tastes and textures in a crunchy, delicious snack.
2 rice cakes per serving
Time for Preparation and Cooking: 5 **minutes**

Ingredients:
- 1 rice cake, 2
- 2 tablespoons of nut butter, such as peanut or almond
- sliced thinly 1 banana
- Chia seeds as an ornament

Instructions:
1. On each rice cake, equally distribute the nut butter.

2. Put a thin layer of banana slices on top of the nut butter.

3. Chia seeds may be added for extra crunch and nutrients.

4. Serve right away and delight in it!

4. Hummus and Veggie Sticks

An explosion of tastes and colors in a light, pleasant snack.

Size of Serving: 1 serving

Time for Preparation and Cooking: 10 **minutes**

Ingredients:

- Banana sticks
- carrot sticks
- sliced bell peppers
- Plum tomatoes

- To dip in hummus

Instructions:

1. Vegetables should be washed and chopped into strips and sticks.

2. Place the vegetables in a serving tray or on a dish.

3. Present hummus on the side for dipping.

4. Enjoy this tasty and healthy snack!

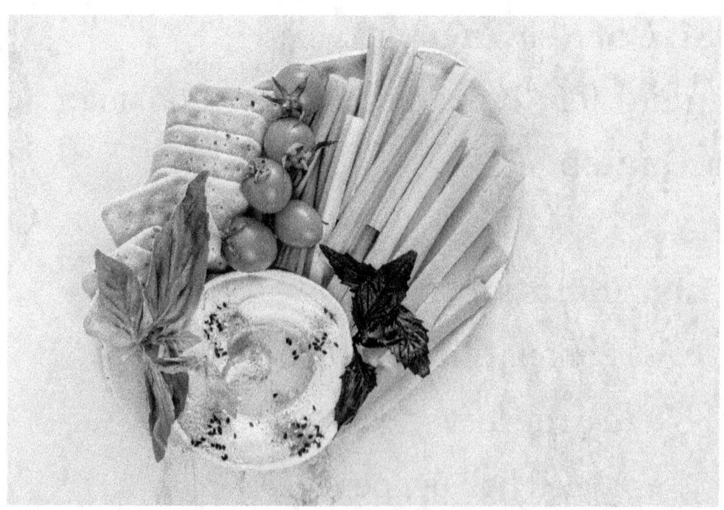

5. Chickpeas Roasted

A protein-rich snack of crunchy and flavorful roasted chickpeas.

Size of serving: 1/2 cup

Cooking and preparation time: **40 minutes**

Ingredients:

- 1 can (15 oz) washed and drained chickpeas
- Olive oil, 1 tbsp
- 1 paprika teaspoon
- 1/8 tsp. cumin
- pepper and salt as desired

Instructions:

1. Set the oven's temperature to 400°F (200°C).

2. The chickpeas should be well-dried before adding spices and olive oil.

3. On a baking sheet, spread them out, and bake for 30-35 minutes, or until crispy.

4. For a crispy snack, allow them to cool and store in an airtight container.

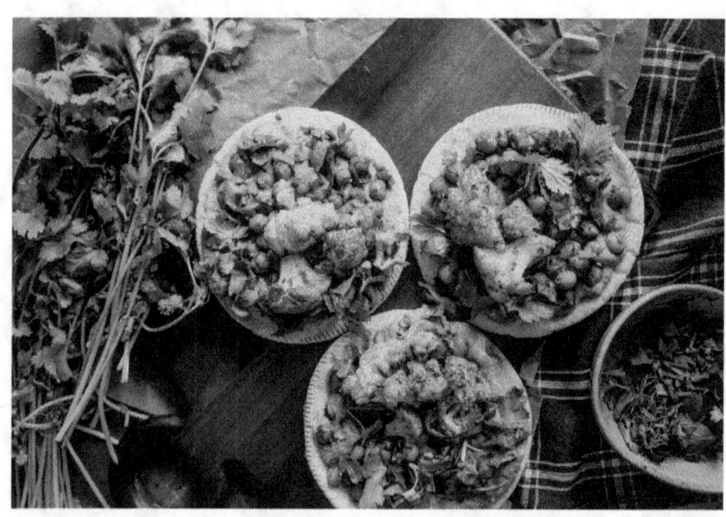

6. Slices of apple with almond butter

A straightforward snack that's healthy and has a satisfying crunch.

Slices of an apple's worth of servings

Time for Preparation and Cooking: **5 minutes**

Ingredients:

- 1 finely sliced apple
- Almond butter, two teaspoons
- a dash of cinnamon

Instructions:

1. The apple should be cleaned and thinly sliced.
2. Each slice should have almond butter on it.

3. Add some cinnamon to the mix for taste.

4. Place the pieces on a dish, then indulge!

7. Cups for quinoa salad

A compact, bite-sized protein-rich snack in quinoa cups.

Size of Serving: 3 cups

Cooking and preparation time: **25 minutes**

Ingredients:

- cooked quinoa, 1 cup
- 1/2 cup washed and drained black beans
- 14 cup chopped cherry tomatoes
- diced 1/4 cup cucumber
- freshly cut parsley

- Juice of lemon, if desired

- pepper and salt as desired

Instructions:

1. Set the oven's temperature to 350°F (175°C).

2. Quinoa, black beans, cherry tomatoes, cucumber, and parsley should all be combined in a dish.

3. Mix thoroughly before adding lemon juice, salt, and pepper to taste.

4. Place the mixture in a tiny muffin pan that has been prepared and bake for 15-20 minutes.

5. Before taking them from the tin, let them cool, then serve and savor!

8. Spinach and Egg Mini Muffins

Muffins that are loaded with protein and healthy ingredients like eggs and spinach.

Size of Serving: 2 tiny muffins

Cooking and preparation time: **25 minutes**

Ingredients:

- 4 eggs
- chopped spinach leaves from a half-cup
- pepper and salt as desired

Instructions:

1. Grease a small muffin tray and preheat the oven to 350°F (175°C).
2. Beat the eggs in a bowl and stir in the spinach, salt, and pepper.
3. Fill the muffin tray with the mixture.

4. Bake the muffins for 15-20 minutes, or until they are done.

5. Remove from the tin after cooling, then enjoy!

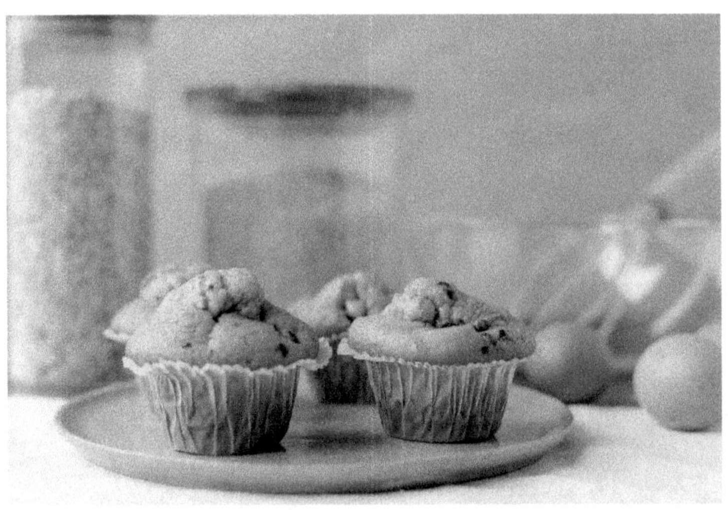

9. Path Mix

A customizable combination of nuts and dried fruits for an instant energy boost.

Size of Serving: 1/4 cup

Time for Preparation and Cooking: **5 minutes**

Ingredients:
- Almonds
- Walnuts
- Dehydrated cranberries
- chopped dried apricots
- black chocolate chips

Instructions:
1. In a bowl, combine the desired quantities of each ingredient.

2. For a quick snack, keep the trail mix in
an airtight container.

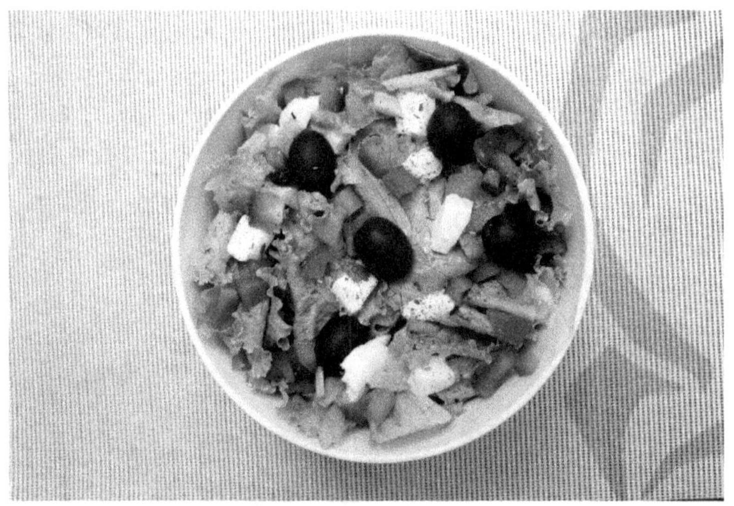

10. Skewers of cottage cheese with pineapple

An energizing and protein-packed snack on skewers.

Size of Serving: two skewers

Time for Preparation and Cooking: **10 minutes**

Ingredients:

- cubes of cottage cheese
- pieces of fresh pineapple
- toothpicks or skewers

Instructions:

1. Each skewer or toothpick should include a pineapple chunk first, then a bit of cottage cheese.
2. Do this for each skewer.
3. Serve these spicy and sweet skewers as a tasty snack!

RECIPES FOR APPETIZER

1. Spicy Avocado Salsa

Brief Summary/Background: A tangy salsa that is full of flavor and good fats is ideal for pre-workout eating.

4 servings per item.

Ten minutes for cooking and preparation

Ingredients:

- 2 diced ripe avocados, 1 diced tomato, 1/2 finely chopped red onion, and 1 minced jalapeno
- 1 lime's worth of juice, diced 1/4 cup fresh cilantro
- pepper and salt as desired

Step-by-Step Guidelines

1. Combine the avocados, tomato, red onion, jalapeno, and cilantro gently in a medium bowl.
2. Season the mixture with salt & pepper and lime juice. Mix thoroughly.
3. Serve right away with veggie sticks or whole-wheat tortilla chips.

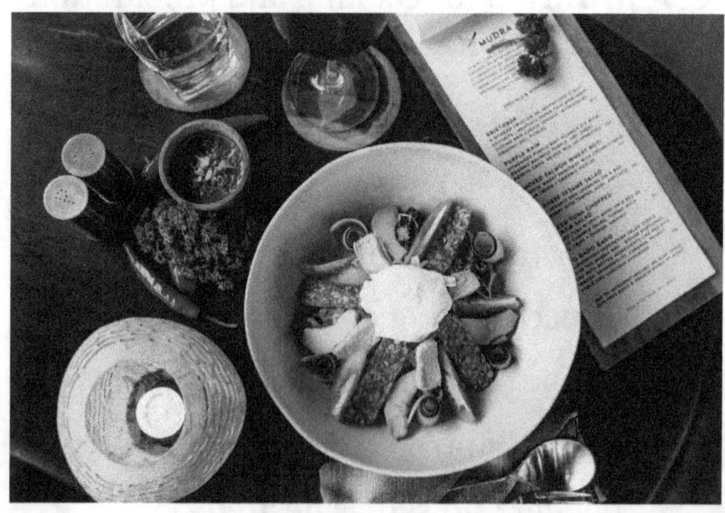

2. Sweet Potato Wedges Baked

Brief Description/Background: These wedges are perfectly seasoned and baked for a delightful crunch, making them a guilt-free substitute for traditional fries.

Two servings per recipe

30-minute preparation and cooking time

Ingredients:

- wedges sliced from two medium sweet potatoes that have been rinsed
- Olive oil, 1 tbsp
- 1 paprika teaspoon
- 1 teaspoon of powdered garlic
- pepper and salt as desired

Step-by-Step Guidelines

1. The oven should be heated to 400°F (200°C).

2. Sweet potato wedges should be equally coated in a bowl with olive oil, paprika, garlic powder, salt, and pepper.

3. Place the wedges in a single layer on a baking sheet, and bake for 25 to 30 minutes, or until crispy and golden.

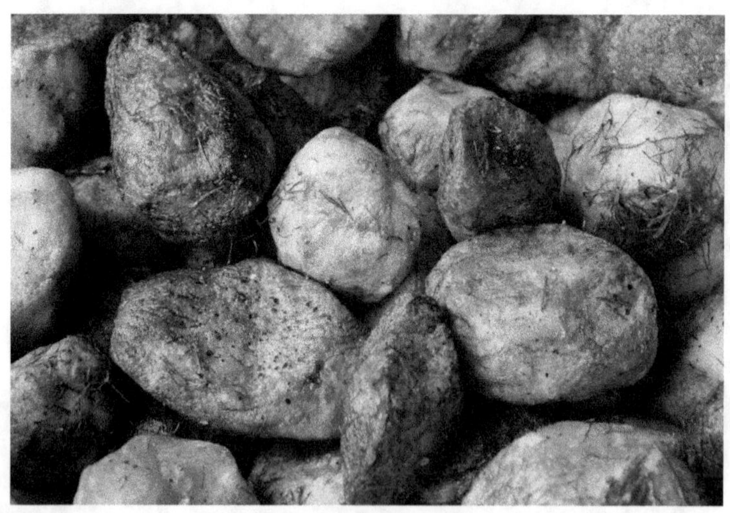

3. Quinoa-stuffed mushrooms

A protein-rich, nutrient-rich appetizer that is tasty and filling is the perfect pre-dinner snack, according to the brief description or backstory.

Serving Size: 6 servings, each with 2 mushrooms

Duration of preparation and cooking: **35 minutes**

Ingredients:

- stems cut off of 12 big mushroom caps and neatly chopped
- 1/2 cup cooked and rinsed quinoa
- 14 cup finely chopped onion
- 14 cups coarsely chopped red bell pepper
- 1 minced garlic clove

- grated Parmesan cheese, 1/4 cup
- garnishing with fresh parsley
- pepper and salt as desired

Step-by-Step Guidelines

1. The oven should be heated to 375°F (190°C).
2. Mushroom stems, red bell pepper, onion, and garlic should all be cooked until soft in a pan.
3. Combine the sautéed mixture, cooked quinoa, and Parmesan cheese in a bowl. Add salt and pepper to taste.
4. Place the mushroom caps on a baking sheet and fill with the quinoa mixture.
5. Bake the mushrooms for 15 to 20 minutes, or until they are soft.
6. Before serving, garnish with fresh parsley.

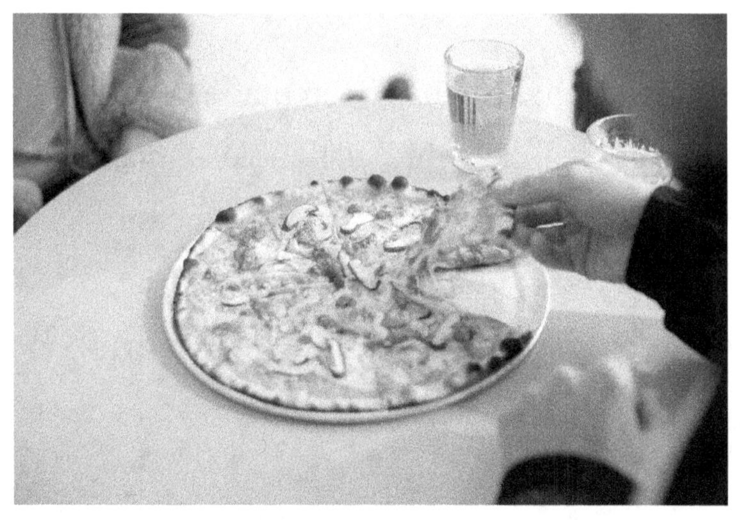

125

4. Artichoke and Spinach Dip

A traditional dip has been made healthier by adding spinach and artichokes, making it the ideal light treat before working out.

4 servings per item.

Cooking and preparation time: 25 minutes

Ingredients:

- 1 box (10 ounces) of thawed and drained frozen chopped spinach
- 1 (14-ounce) can of chopped and drained artichoke hearts
- Greek yogurt, half a cup
- Light mayonnaise, 1/4 cup
- grated Parmesan cheese, 1/4 cup
- Shredded mozzarella cheese in a cup
- 1 minced garlic clove

- pepper and salt as desired

Step-by-Step Guidelines

1. The oven should be heated to 375°F (190°C).

2. Spinach, artichokes, Greek yogurt, mayonnaise, Parmesan cheese, mozzarella cheese, and garlic are all combined in a bowl. Mix thoroughly.

3. Once the mixture has been seasoned with salt and pepper, put it in a baking dish.

4. Bake for 15 to 20 minutes, or until the top is bubbling and gently brown.

5. Serve hot with veggie sticks or whole-wheat pita chips.

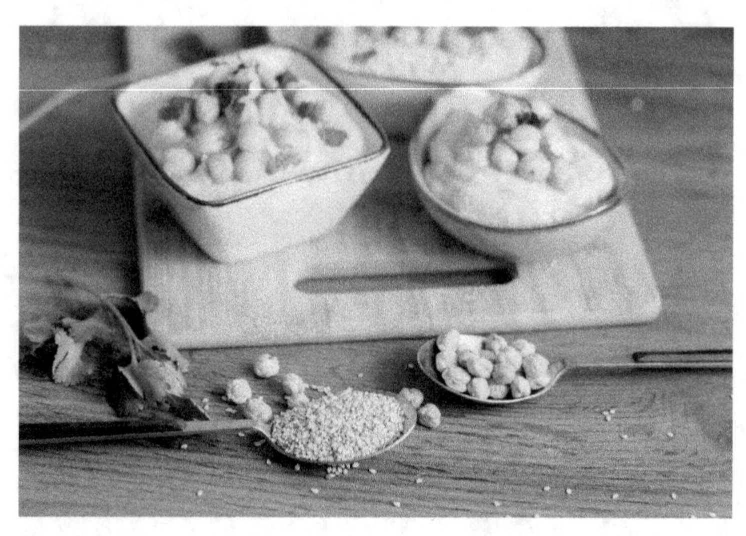

5. Chickpea Hummus with Protein

Brief Description/Background: A high-protein, satiating snack prepared from chickpeas that promotes muscle repair.

6 servings per item.

15 minutes for cooking and preparation

Ingredients:

- 1 can (15 ounces) of rinsed and drained chickpeas
- Tahini, 14 cup
- Olive oil, 1/4 cup
- lemon juice from one
- 2 minced garlic cloves
- 1 teaspoon of cumin, ground
- Water (as required to achieve desired consistency) Salt & pepper to taste

Step-by-Step Guidelines

1. Blend the following ingredients in a food processor: chickpeas, tahini, olive oil, lemon juice, garlic, cumin, salt, and pepper.
2. To reach the required creamy consistency, gradually add water.
3. If necessary, taste and adjust the seasoning.
4. Before serving, transfer to a serving dish and top with a little olive oil.

6. Turkey and Quinoa Stuffed Bell Peppers

Brief Synopsis/Background: These protein-rich bell peppers are filled with a healthy mixture of quinoa and lean turkey, making them the perfect appetizer.

Serving Size: 4 servings, each with a stuffed pepper.

Cooking and preparation time: 45 minutes

Ingredients:

- 4 bell peppers, seeded and cut in half
- 1/2 cup cooked and rinsed quinoa
- Half a pound of lean ground turkey and a cup of finely chopped onion
- 1 minced garlic clove
- 50 ml of tomato sauce

- Shredded mozzarella cheese in a cup
- pepper and salt as desired

Step-by-Step Guidelines

1. The oven should be heated to 375°F (190°C).

2. Put the cut-side up in a baking tray with the bell pepper halves.

3. Cook the ground turkey, onion, and garlic in a pan until the meat is browned and well-cooked.

7. Veggie sticks and Greek Tzatziki

Brief Synopsis/Background: For a healthy and energizing pre-workout snack, fresh vegetable sticks are coupled with a creamy and tangy Greek yogurt dip.

4 servings per item.

Ten minutes for cooking and preparation

Ingredients:

- Greek yogurt, one cup
- Finely chopped and drained half a cucumber
- 2 minced garlic cloves
- 1 tablespoon finely sliced fresh dill
- lemon juice from one
- pepper and salt as desired
- Various vegetable sticks for dipping (cucumbers, carrots, and bell peppers)

Step-by-Step Guidelines

1. Greek yogurt, grated cucumber, garlic, dill, lemon juice, salt, and pepper should all be combined in a bowl. Mix thoroughly.
2. With a dish of veggie sticks, serve cold.

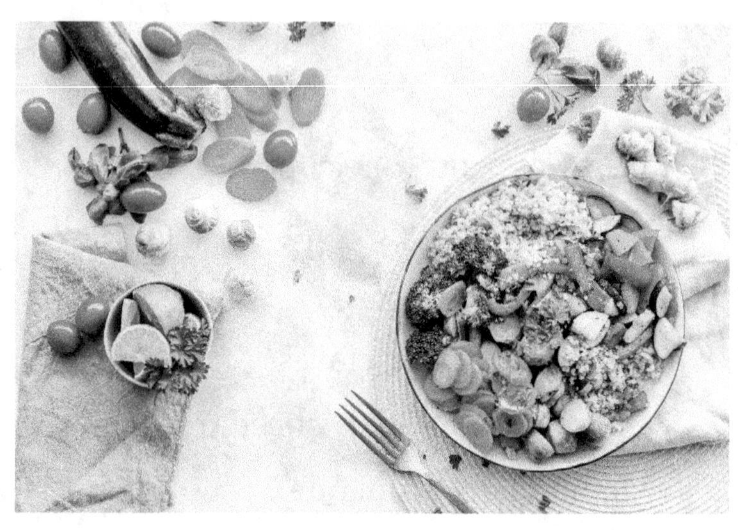

8. Baked Parmesan Zucchini Chips

Brief Description/Background: Crispy, Parmesan-coated zucchini chips cooked in the oven provide a low-carb, guilt-free appetizer.

4 servings per item.

Cooking and preparation time: 25 minutes

Ingredients:

- 2 big, thinly sliced zucchini
- grated Parmesan cheese, half a cup
- one-half teaspoon of garlic powder
- a half-teaspoon of dried oregano
- Taste-tested salt and pepper Cooking spray

Step-by-Step Guidelines

1. Set a baking sheet on the counter and preheat the oven to 425°F (220°C).

2. Parmesan cheese, garlic powder, dried oregano, salt, and pepper should all be combined in a bowl.

3. Slices of zucchini are placed on the baking pan after being coated on both sides with the cheese mixture.

4. Spray some cooking spray on the slices sparingly.

5. Bake the chips for 15 to 20 minutes, or until crisp and golden.

9. Spicy Edamame

Brief Summary/Background: This recipe for spicy, protein-rich edamame is ideal for individuals who want a little spice with their appetizers.

4 servings per item.

15 minutes for cooking and preparation

Ingredients:

- 2 cups thawed frozen edamame
- Olive oil, two teaspoons
- one tablespoon of chili powder
- a half-teaspoon of smoked paprika
- Salt as desired

Step-by-Step Guidelines

1. Olive oil is heated over medium-high heat in a pan.

2. Add the frozen edamame and cook for three to five minutes.

3. Salt, smoked paprika, and chili powder should be added to the edamame. A good stir will coat.

4. Sauté the edamame for a further 2 to 3 minutes, or until it is cooked through and beginning to become crispy.

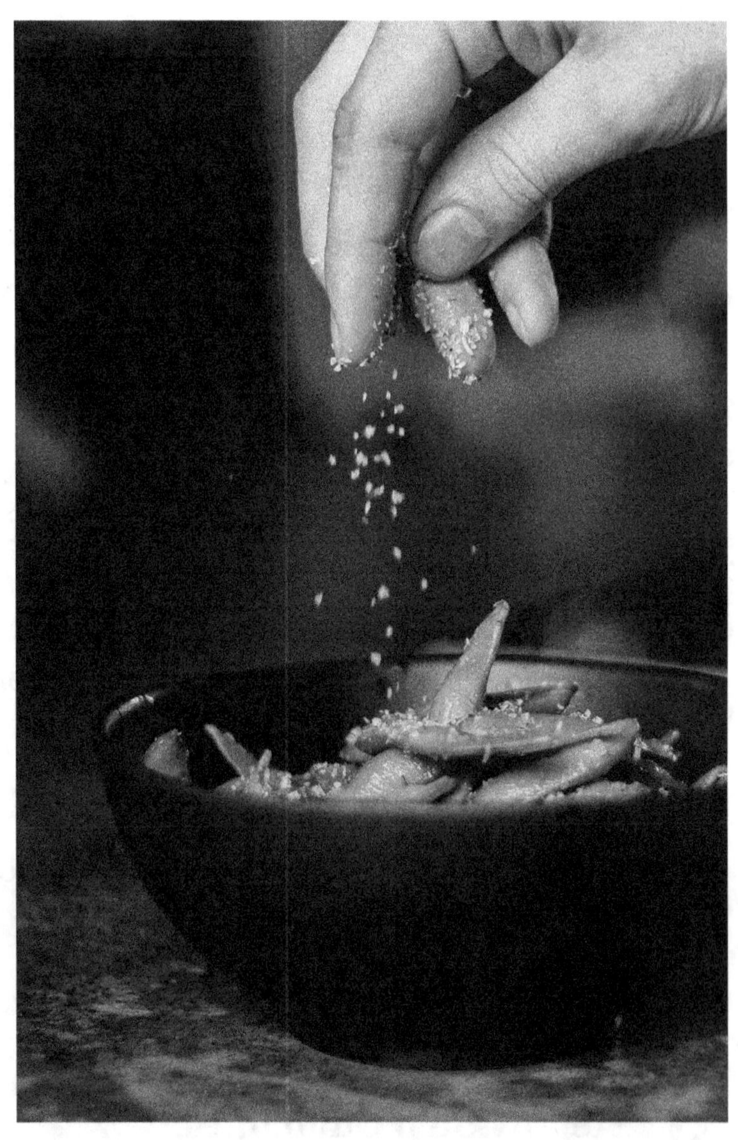

10. Caprese Skewers

Short Description/Background: A simple but sophisticated snack made with the traditional Caprese ingredients of fresh mozzarella, cherry tomatoes, and basil.

Servings Per Recipe: 4

15 minutes for preparation and cooking

Substances:

- 12 cherry tomatoes - 12 bocconcini, which are little balls of fresh mozzarella - 12 sprigs of fresh basil - drizzled balsamic vinegar - wooden skewers
- To taste, salt and pepper

Step-by-Step Guidelines:

1. Wrap a basil leaf, a mozzarella ball, and a cherry tomato around each wooden skewer.

2. When you have 12 skewers, repeat step 2.

3. Just before serving, arrange the skewers on a dish, season with salt and pepper, and drizzle with the balsamic glaze.

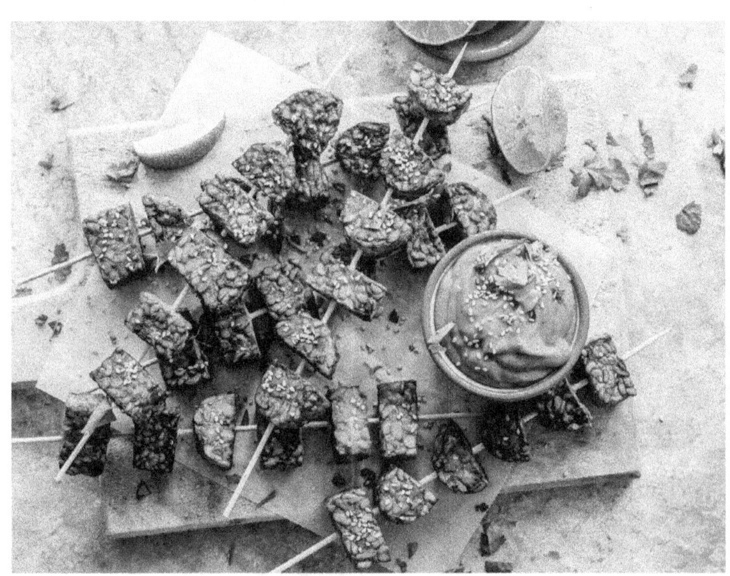

1. Tropical Paradise Smoothie

With this hydrating and healthy smoothie, take a trip to the tropics.

Two servings per recipe

Cooking and preparation time: 5 minutes

Ingredients:

- 1 cup of pieces of fresh pineapple
- one ripe banana
- Coconut milk, half a cup
- Greek yogurt, half a cup
- Honey, 1 tablespoon
- Ice cubes, if desired

Instructions:

1. Blend all the ingredients.

2. Until smooth, blend.

3. If desired, add ice cubes and mix one more.

4. Pour into cups, then sip.

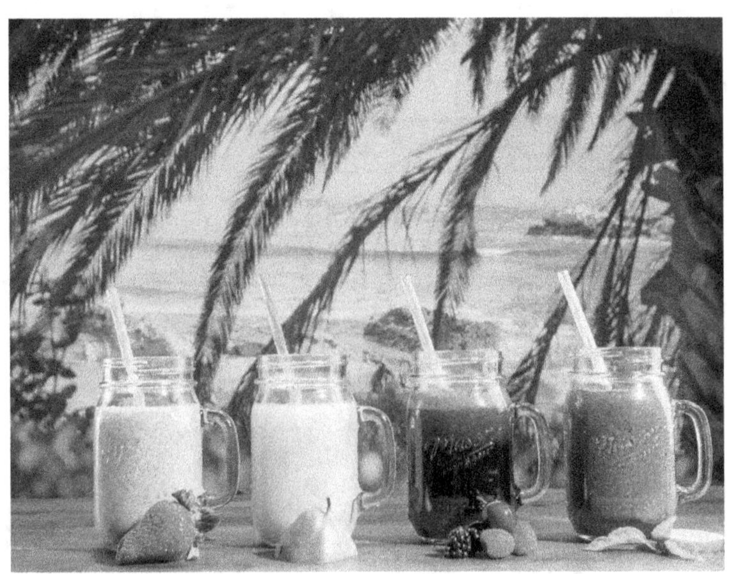

2. Smoothie with Berry Blast

A colorful combination of berries for an antioxidant boost.

Two servings per recipe

Cooking and preparation time: 5 minutes

Ingredients:

- strawberries, blueberries, and raspberries in a cup
- Vanilla yogurt, half a cup
- Almond milk, half a cup
- Honey, 1 tablespoon
- Vanilla extract, half a teaspoon

Instructions:

1. In a blender, combine all the ingredients.

2. Until smooth, blend.

3. If necessary, taste and add additional honey.

4. Pour into glasses, then savor the delicious berry flavor.

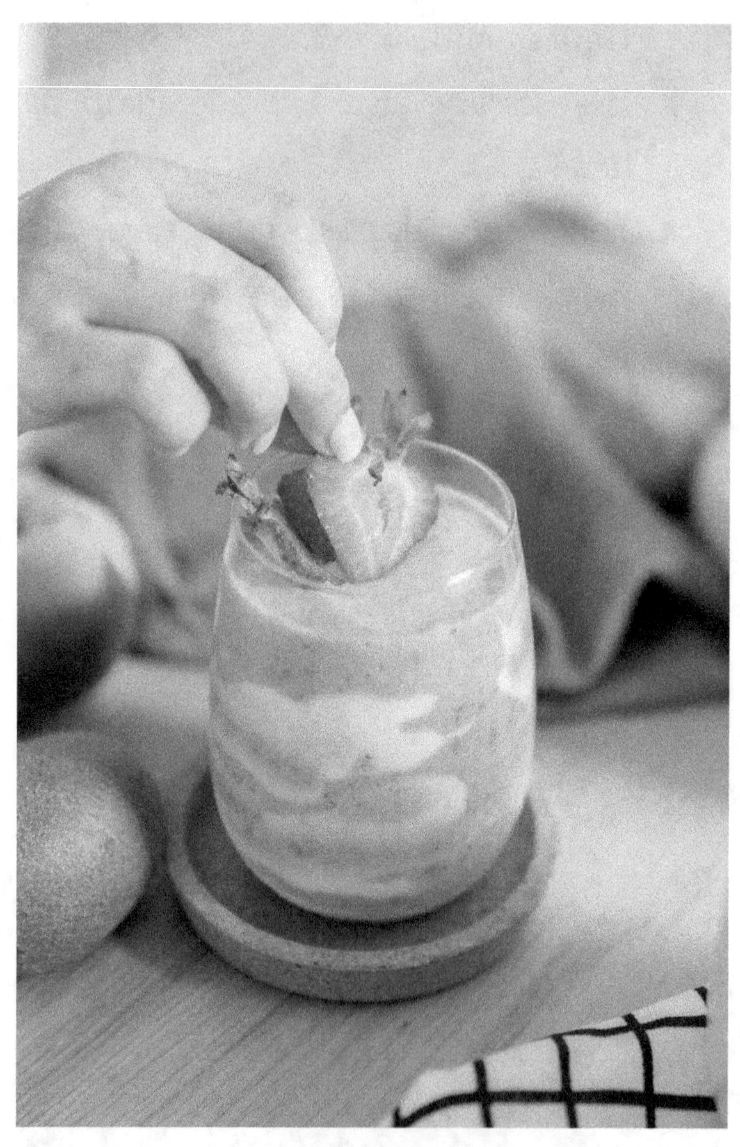

3. A green smoothie.

A green smoothie that is filled with nutrients to start your day.

Size of Serving: 1 serving

Cooking and preparation time: 7 minutes

Ingredients:

- spinach leaves, 1 cup
- 12 an avocado
- half a banana
- Unsweetened almond milk in 1/2 cup
- Chia seeds, 1 tbsp
- 1 teaspoon of optional honey

Instructions:

1. In a blender, combine spinach, avocado, banana, almond milk, and chia seeds.
2. Until smooth, blend.
3. If desired, add honey for sweetness.
4. Pour into a glass, then enjoy your jolt of green energy!

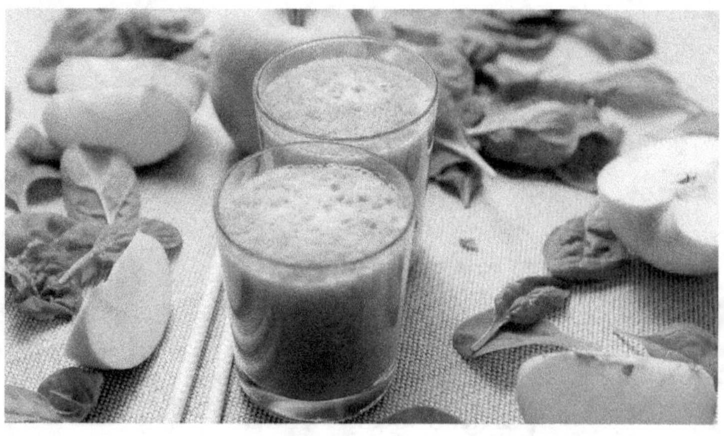

4. Protein Shake with Peanut Butter

A smoothie filled with protein for post-workout recovery.

Size of Serving: 1 serving

Cooking and preparation time: 5 minutes

Ingredients:

- one banana
- Peanut butter, two teaspoons
- 1 cup of milk, either dairy or vegan
- 1 scoop of protein powder in vanilla
- Cinnamon, half a teaspoon
- Ice cubes, if desired

Instructions:

1. In a blender, combine the banana, peanut butter, milk, protein powder, and cinnamon.

2. Until smooth, blend.

3. If you want it cooler, add ice cubes and combine once more.

4. Pour your protein-packed shake into a glass, and then sip it.

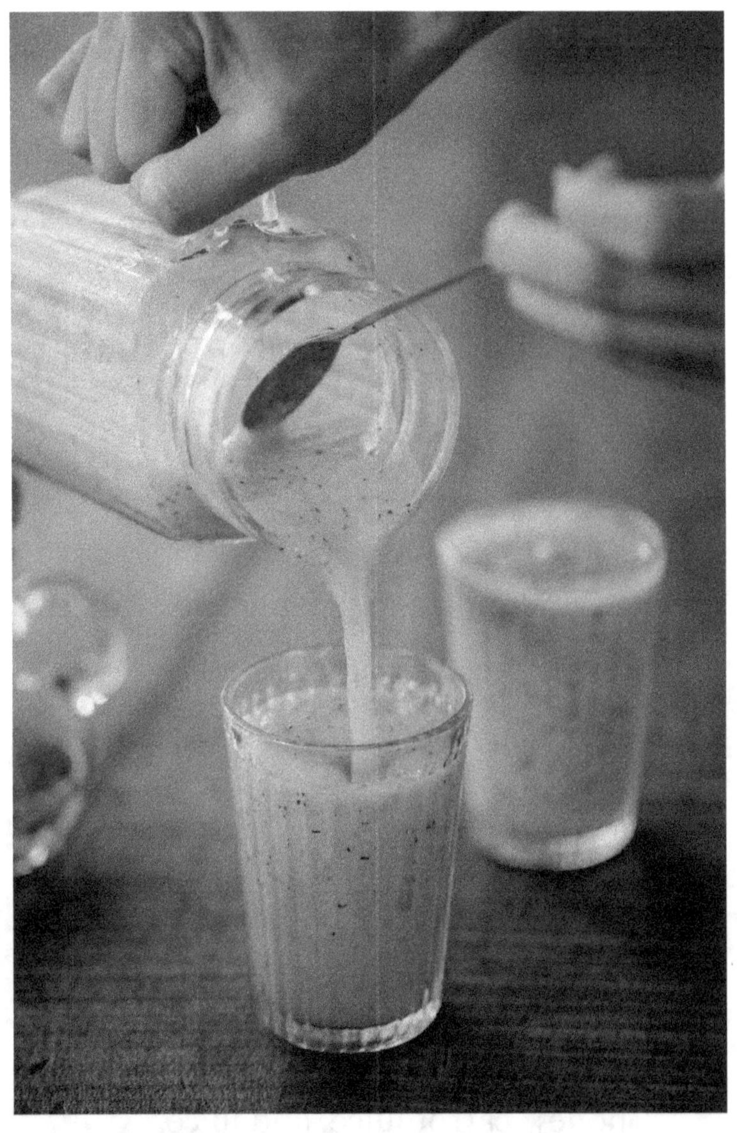

5. Cinnamon Sunrise Smoothie

A tangy and cooling smoothie to start the morning, in brief.

Two servings per recipe

Cooking and preparation time: 5 minutes

Ingredients:

- Segmenting and peeling two oranges
- Greek yogurt, half a cup
- carrot juice in a half-cup
- Honey, 1 tablespoon
- Ice cubes, if desired

Instructions:

1. Blend oranges with Greek yogurt, honey, carrot juice, and juice.
2. Until smooth, blend.

3. If desired, add ice cubes and mix one more.

4. Pour into glasses, then sip on the sunlight!

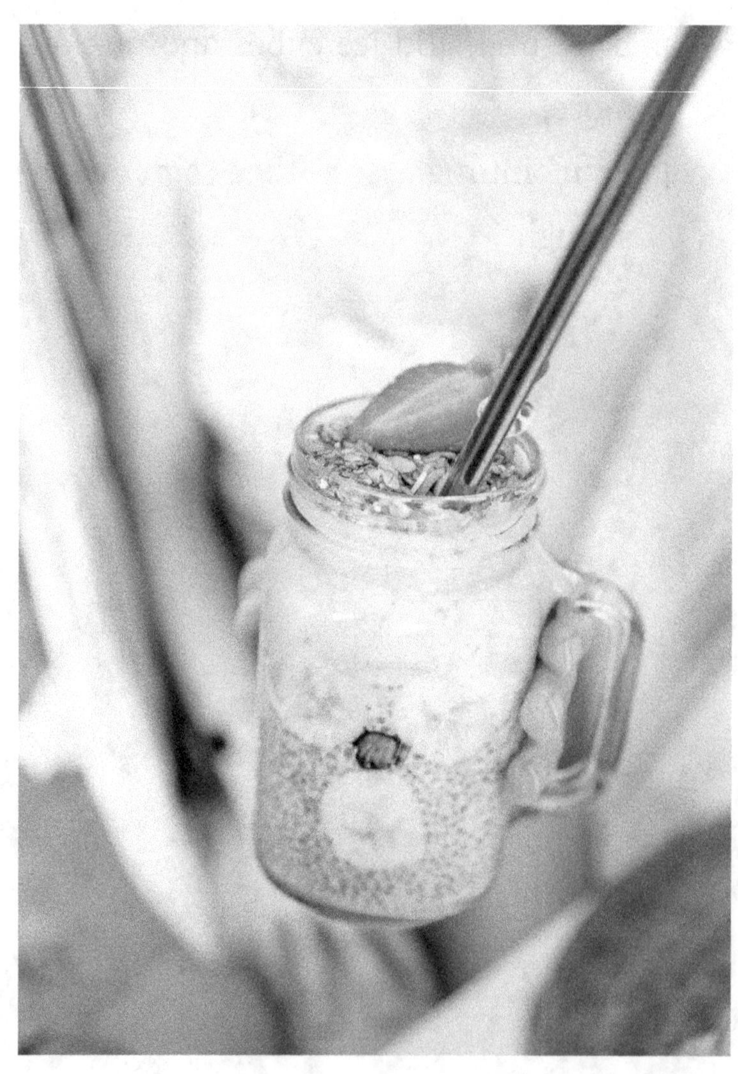

6. Choco-Banana Smoothie

A smoothie that is creamy and decadent with a dash of chocolate.

Two servings per recipe

Cooking and preparation time: 5 minutes

Ingredients:

- two ripe bananas
- Cocoa powder, 2 teaspoons
- 1 cup of milk, either dairy or vegan
- Greek yogurt, half a cup
- Honey, 1 tablespoon

Instructions:

1. Blend milk, Greek yogurt, honey, ripe bananas, chocolate powder, and other ingredients in a blender.

2. Until smooth, blend.

3. If desired, taste and add extra honey.

4. Pour the chocolate banana pleasure into glasses and enjoy.

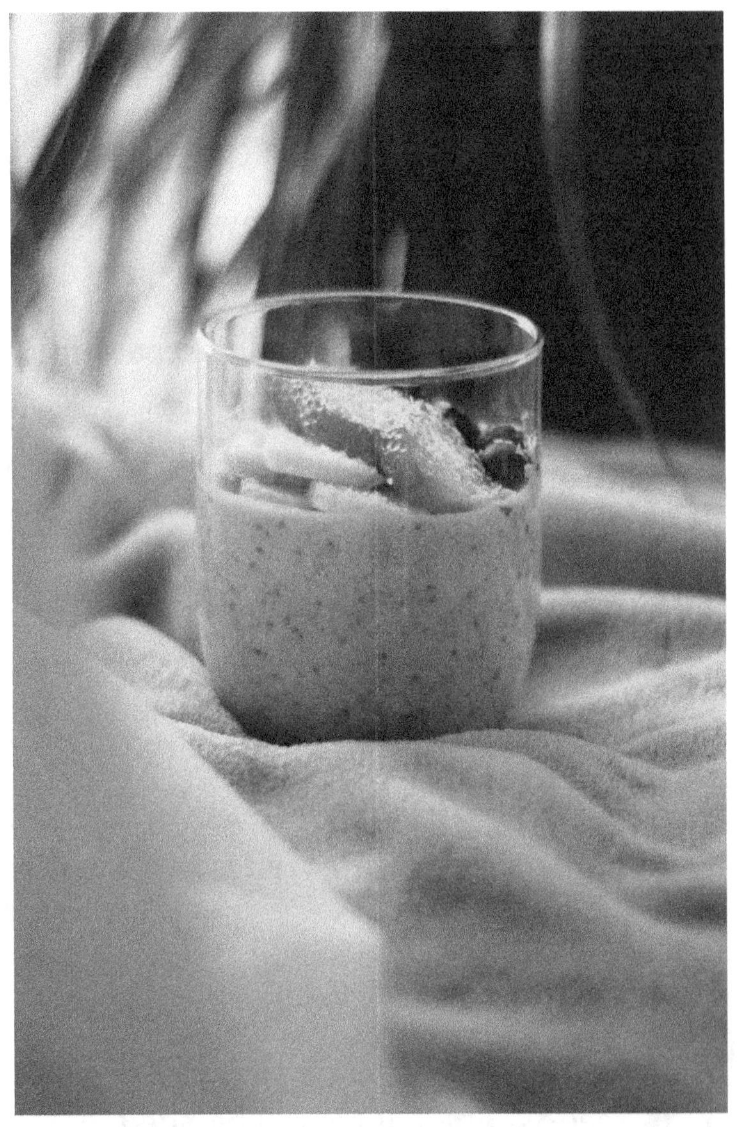

7. Green Superfood Smoothie Bowl

A richer, superfood-filled variant of the green smoothie served in a bowl.

Size of Serving: 1 bowl

Ten minutes for cooking and preparation

Ingredients:

- Greens from 1 cup of kale
- Frozen mixed berries in a cup
- 12 an avocado
- Chia seeds, 1 tbsp
- Granola, 1/4 cup
- Banana slices with berries as a garnish

Instructions:

1. Kale, frozen berries, avocado, and chia seeds should all be well blended.
2. Put some in a bowl.

3. Add granola, banana slices, and berries as garnish.

4. With a spoon, enjoy your healthy green smoothie bowl!

8. Smoothie with creamy almond joy

A delicious combination of almond, coconut, and chocolate tastes.

Two servings per recipe

Cooking and preparation time: 5 minutes

Ingredients:

- Unsweetened almond butter in 1/2 cup
- two teaspoons of coconut shreds
- Cocoa powder, 2 teaspoons
- Almond milk in two cups
- 1/4 cup of almond slices
- Ice cubes, if desired

Instructions:

1. Blend almond butter, coconut shreds, cocoa nibs, almond milk, and ice cubes in a blender.

2. Until smooth, blend.

3. Enjoy your creamy almond bliss by pouring it into glasses and topping them with sliced almonds.

9. Smoothie with oatmeal cookies

The flavor of oatmeal cookies is in the shape of a healthy smoothie.

Two servings per recipe

Cooking and preparation time: 5 minutes

Ingredients:

- Rollin oats in a cup, half
- one ripe banana
- Almond butter, two teaspoons
- Cinnamon, half a teaspoon
- 1 cup of milk, either dairy or vegan
- Ice cubes, if desired

Instructions:

1. Blend the rolled oats, milk, ice cubes, almond butter, cinnamon, and ripe banana in a blender.

2. Until smooth, blend.

3. Pour into glasses and savor the taste of oatmeal cookies that bring back memories.

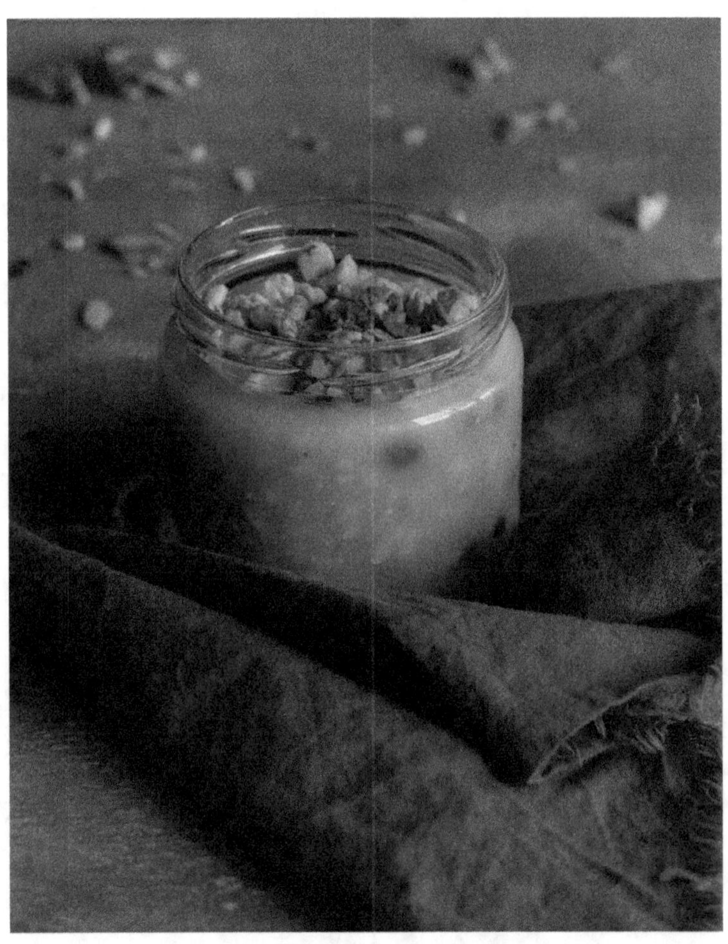

10. Matcha Smoothie with Energy

A smoothie fortified with matcha green tea for a caffeine boost.

Serving Size: One serving

5 minutes for preparation and cooking

Substances:

- Matcha green tea powder, 1 teaspoon
- One banana
- Greek yogurt, 1/2 cup
- 1 spoonful of honey - 1/2 cup of coconut water

Requirements:

1. Mix a little boiling water with the matcha green tea powder, then let it cool.

2. In a blender, combine the matcha mixture with the banana, Greek yogurt, coconut water, and honey.

3. Blend until fluid.

4. Pour your invigorating matcha smoothie into a glass and sip.

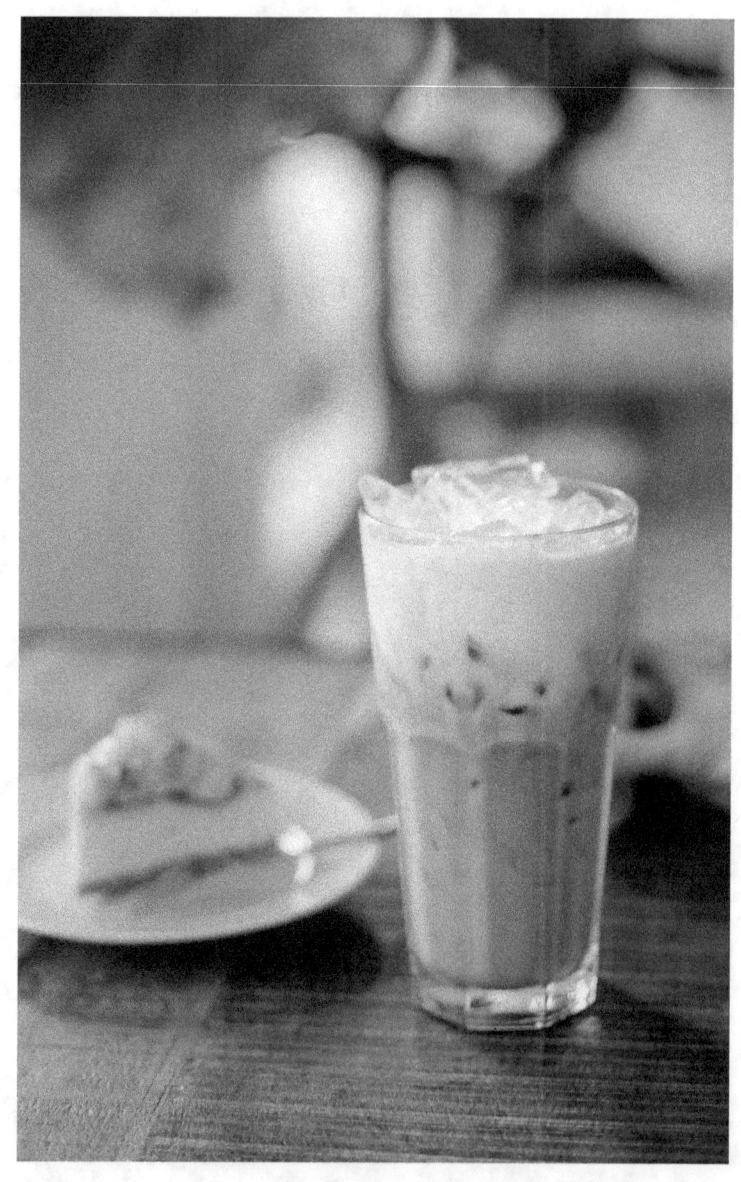

RECIPES FOR SOUP AND SIDE DISHES

1. Cheesy Garlic Bread and Creamy Tomato Basil Soup

For a traditional and filling lunch, handmade cheesy garlic bread is served with this substantial tomato basil soup.

4 servings per item.

30-minute preparation and cooking time

Ingredients:

- Two 28-ounce cans of whole, peeled tomatoes
- 1/2 cup heavy cream and 1 cup vegetable broth
- 14 cup chopped fresh basil leaves

- pepper and salt as desired

- Four French bread slices

- Shredded mozzarella cheese in a cup

- 2 minced garlic cloves

- Butter, two tablespoons

Instructions:

1. The tinned tomatoes and vegetable broth should be combined in a big saucepan. Cook for ten minutes.

2. The tomato mixture should be smooth after being pureed with an immersion blender. Put it back in the pot.

3. Fresh basil and heavy cream should be combined. To taste, add salt and pepper to the food. Ten more minutes of simmering.

4. Preheat the oven's broiler while the soup is boiling.

5. Combine the softened butter and minced garlic in a small bowl. Apply this mixture to the French bread pieces.

6. Over the bread pieces, evenly distribute the shredded mozzarella cheese.

7. On a baking sheet, arrange the bread pieces and broil for 2 to 3 minutes, or until the cheese is bubbling and golden.

8. With a side of cheesy garlic bread, serve the soup hot.

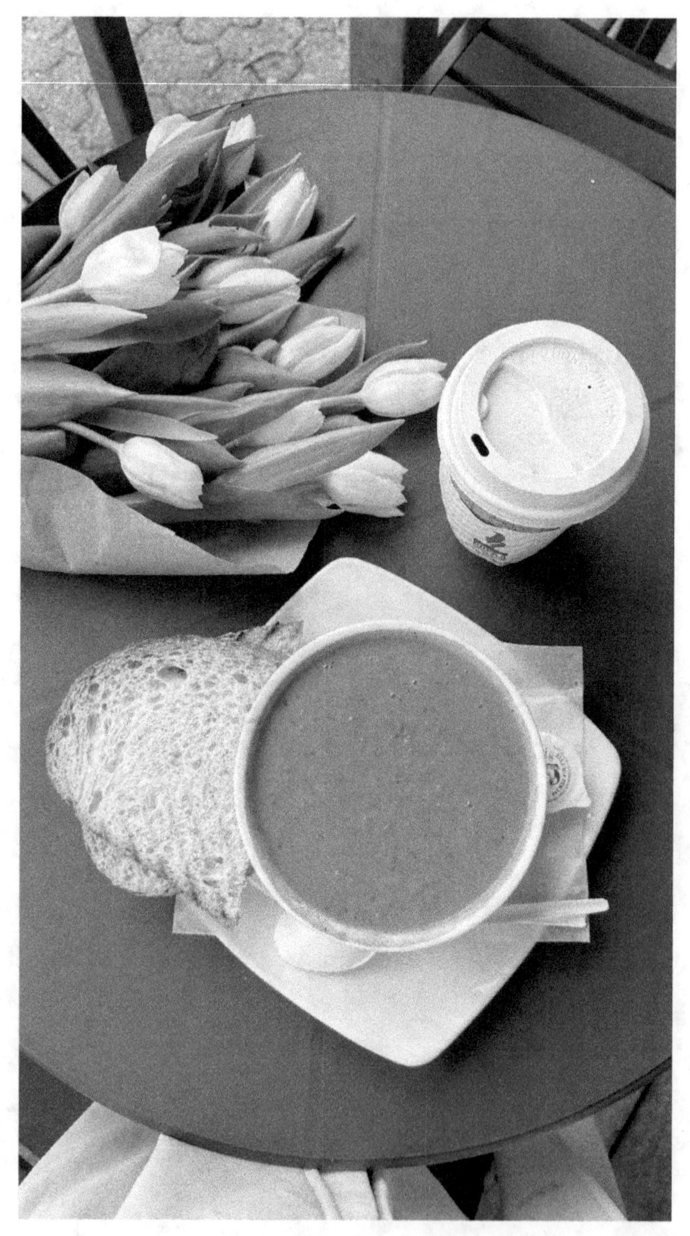

2. Rosemary Parmesan Biscuits with Roasted Butternut Squash Soup

A creamy butternut squash soup coupled with salty rosemary Parmesan cookies is ideal for winter nights, according to the short description.

4 servings per item.

Cooking and preparation time: 45 minutes

Ingredients:

- One medium butternut squash, chopped after being peeled
- 1 diced onion, 2 minced garlic cloves
- 4 cups of veggie broth
- 50 ml of thick cream
- 1 fresh rosemary sprig
- pepper and salt as desired

- 2 cups of general-purpose flour
- 1 teaspoon of baking soda
- 0.5 teaspoons of salt
- grated Parmesan cheese, half a cup
- Cold, cubed, and half a cup of unsalted butter
- 0.5 cups of milk

Instructions:

1. Set the oven's temperature to 400°F (200°C). Roast the diced butternut squash for 25 to 30 minutes, or until it's soft and just beginning to caramelize, on a baking sheet with a sprinkle of olive oil.

2. The chopped onion and garlic should be cooked until transparent in a big saucepan.

3. Vegetable broth and the roasted butternut squash should be added. Cook for 10 minutes after bringing to a simmer.

4. Until the soup is creamy, purée it using an immersion blender. Add fresh rosemary and heavy cream after stirring. Add salt and pepper to taste.

5. For the biscuits, combine the flour, baking soda, salt, and grated Parmesan in a mixing basin.

6. Until the mixture resembles coarse crumbs, gradually include the chilled butter. Add the milk and mix just until incorporated.

7. On a baking sheet, drop spoonfuls of the biscuit dough and bake for 12 to 15 minutes, or until golden brown, at 425°F (220°C).

8. Butternut squash soup should be served with a warm rosemary-parmesan biscuit.

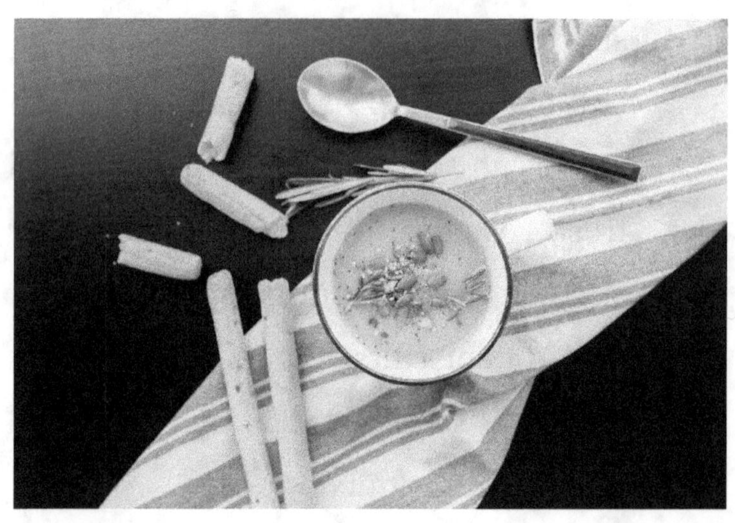

3. Traditional Minestrone Soup with Garlic and Herb Focaccia

A hearty Italian minestrone soup with beans and veggies, served with handmade focaccia topped with garlic and herbs.

6 servings per item.

Cooking and preparation time: 45 minutes

Ingredients:

- 1 cup of carrots, chopped
- 1 cup of celery, diced
- chopped zucchini, 1 cup
- 1 cup washed and drained canned kidney beans
- 1 cup of chopped tomatoes in a can
- 1 cup of little pasta, like ditalini

- 4 cups vegetable broth 2 minced cloves of garlic
- one tablespoon dried basil
- pepper and salt as desired
- Almond oil
- garnishing with fresh parsley

Instructions:

1. Garlic cloves should be minced and sauteed in olive oil until aromatic.
2. Add the chopped zucchini, celery, and carrots. For five minutes, cook.
3. Add the kidney beans, chopped tomatoes, and vegetable broth. Simmer for a while.
4. Pasta and dried basil are combined. Cook the pasta until it is tender.
5. Add salt and pepper to the soup to season it.

6. Slices of garlic herb focaccia should be
   served with the hot dish.

4. Jasmine rice and Thai Coconut Curry.

Thai coconut curry soup that is creamy and flavorful is served with fluffy jasmine rice.

4 servings per item.

30-minute preparation and cooking time

Ingredients:

- One 14-ounce can of coconut milk
- Thai red curry paste, 2 teaspoons, and 2 cups of vegetable broth
- Sliced mushrooms in a cup
- 1 cup of red, yellow, or green bell peppers, thinly sliced
- 1 cup of cooked chicken or tofu diced
- Fish sauce, two teaspoons (for the vegetarian version)
- Brown sugar, 1 tablespoon

- garnish with fresh cilantro
- rice cooked with jasmine

Instructions:

1. Coconut milk, vegetable broth, and red curry paste should all be combined in a big saucepan. Simmer for a while.
2. Add tofu or chicken, as well as mushrooms and bell peppers. Cook the veggies until they are soft.
3. Add brown sugar and fish sauce, if using.
4. Serve the hot Thai coconut curry soup with jasmine rice and fresh cilantro on the side.

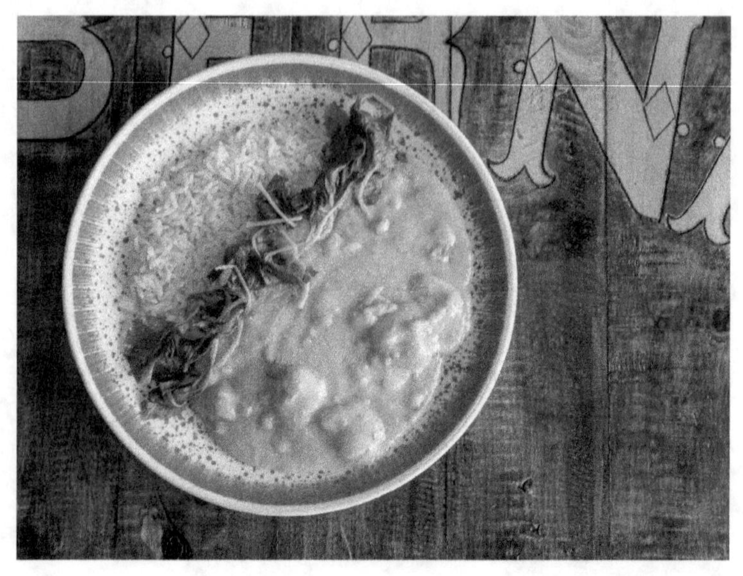

5. Cheddar and chive biscuits with potato-leek soup

A hearty supper of savory cheddar and chive biscuits is served with a creamy potato leek soup.

4 servings per item.

Cooking and preparation time: 40 minutes

Ingredients:

- 4 big potatoes, diced after being peeled
- 2 cleaned and sliced leeks
- 4 cups of veggie broth
- a cup of milk
- To taste, add salt and white pepper.
- 2 cups of general-purpose flour
- 1 teaspoon of baking soda

- 0.5 teaspoons of salt
- grated cheddar cheese, half a cup
- 2 teaspoons chopped fresh chives
- Cold, cubed, and half a cup of unsalted butter

Instructions:

1. Combine potatoes, leeks, and vegetable broth in a big saucepan. Till potatoes are soft, simmer.

2. Until the soup is creamy, purée it using an immersion blender. Add the milk and season with white pepper and salt.

3. For the biscuits, combine the flour, baking soda, salt, shredded cheddar cheese, and chives in a mixing basin.

4. Until the mixture resembles coarse crumbs, gradually include the chilled butter.

5. On a baking sheet, drop spoonfuls of the biscuit dough and bake at 425°F (220°C) for 12 to 15 minutes, or until golden brown.

6. Serve the warm cheddar and chive biscuits with the hot potato leek soup.

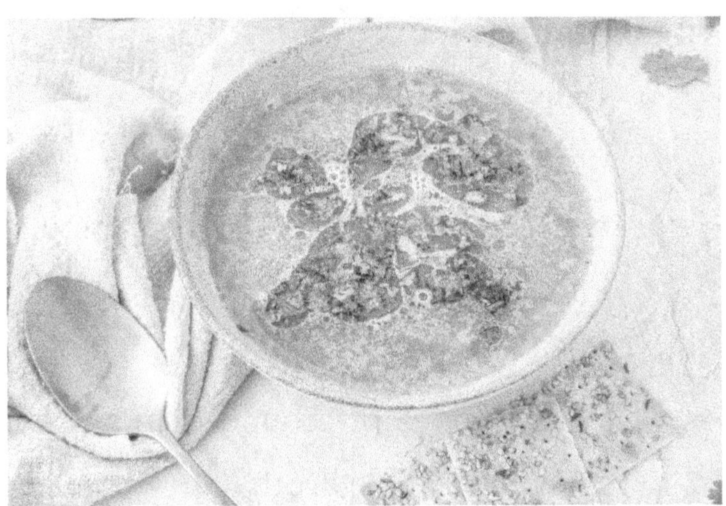

6. Multigrain Bread with Lentil and Veggie Soup

Slices of robust multigrain bread are served with a filling lentil and vegetable soup.

6 servings per item.

Cooking and preparation time: 45 minutes

Ingredients:

- 1 cup of drained and washed green or brown lentils
- two carrots, two celery stalks, and one onion, chopped
- Diced tomatoes, 1 cup
- 2 tablespoons of ground cumin per 6 cups of vegetable broth
- 1 paprika teaspoon
- pepper and salt as desired

- Multigrain bread slices

Instructions:

1. The chopped onion, carrots, and celery should be softened in a big saucepan.
2. Salt, pepper, ground cumin, paprika, chopped tomatoes, vegetable broth, and lentils should all be added. up to a boil.
3. Lentils should be cooked for 25 to 30 minutes on a low heat setting.
4. Slices of multigrain bread should be served with the hot lentil and vegetable soup.

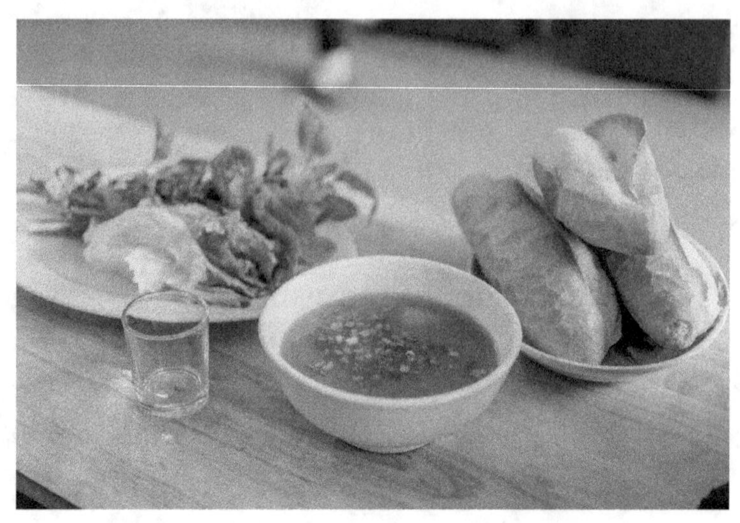

7. Cornbread with Chicken and Wild Rice Soup

Brief Description: Warm, buttery cornbread served with a substantial chicken and wild rice soup.

4 servings per item.

1 hour for preparation and cooking

Ingredients:

- 2 cooked and chopped chicken breasts
- 1 cup cooked wild rice
- two carrots, two celery stalks, and one onion, chopped
- 1 cup milk and 4 cups of chicken broth
- 50 ml of thick cream
- pepper and salt as desired
- cornmeal, 1 cup
- all-purpose flour, 1 cup

- Baking powder and two teaspoons of sugar
- 0.5 teaspoons of salt
- Melted half a cup of unsalted butter
- 2 eggs

Instructions:

1. The chopped onion, carrots, and celery should be softened in a big saucepan.
2. Add the cooked wild rice, milk, heavy cream, chicken broth, and chopped up chicken. Add salt and pepper to taste. For 15 to 20 minutes, simmer.
3. Preheat the oven to 425°F (220°C) for the cornbread. Butter a baking pan.
4. Cornmeal, flour, sugar, baking soda, and salt should all be combined in a mixing dish.

5. Melted butter and eggs should be whisked together in another basin. Stirring is necessary to blend the dry components with this mixture.

6. Fill the baking dish with the cornbread batter, and bake for 20 to 25 minutes, or until golden brown.

7. Slices of warm cornbread should be served with the hot chicken and wild rice soup.

8.   Quiche with spinach and mushrooms and mixed greens

A savory quiche with mushrooms and spinach is served with a light mixed greens salad.

4 servings per item.

Cooking and preparation time: one hour and fifteen minutes

Ingredients:

- 1 prepared pie crust
- 1 cup chopped fresh spinach and 1 cup sliced mushrooms
- shredded Gruyère cheese, half a cup
- Four big eggs
- a cup of milk
- Mixed greens salad with vinaigrette dressing, with salt and pepper to taste

Instructions:

1. Set the oven's temperature to 375°F (190°C). Set aside the pie crust in a pie plate.

2. Sliced mushrooms should be sautéed in a pan until they release moisture and soften. When the spinach has wilted, add the chopped spinach.

3. In the pie crust, distribute the mushroom and spinach mixture equally. Gruyère cheese, grated, should be added on top.

4. Whisk the eggs, milk, salt, and pepper in a bowl. Over the cheese, spinach, and mushrooms, pour this mixture.

5. The quiche should be baked for 35 to 40 minutes, or until the top is brown and the middle is set.

6. Warm spinach and mushroom quiche should be served with a mixed greens salad dressed with vinaigrette.

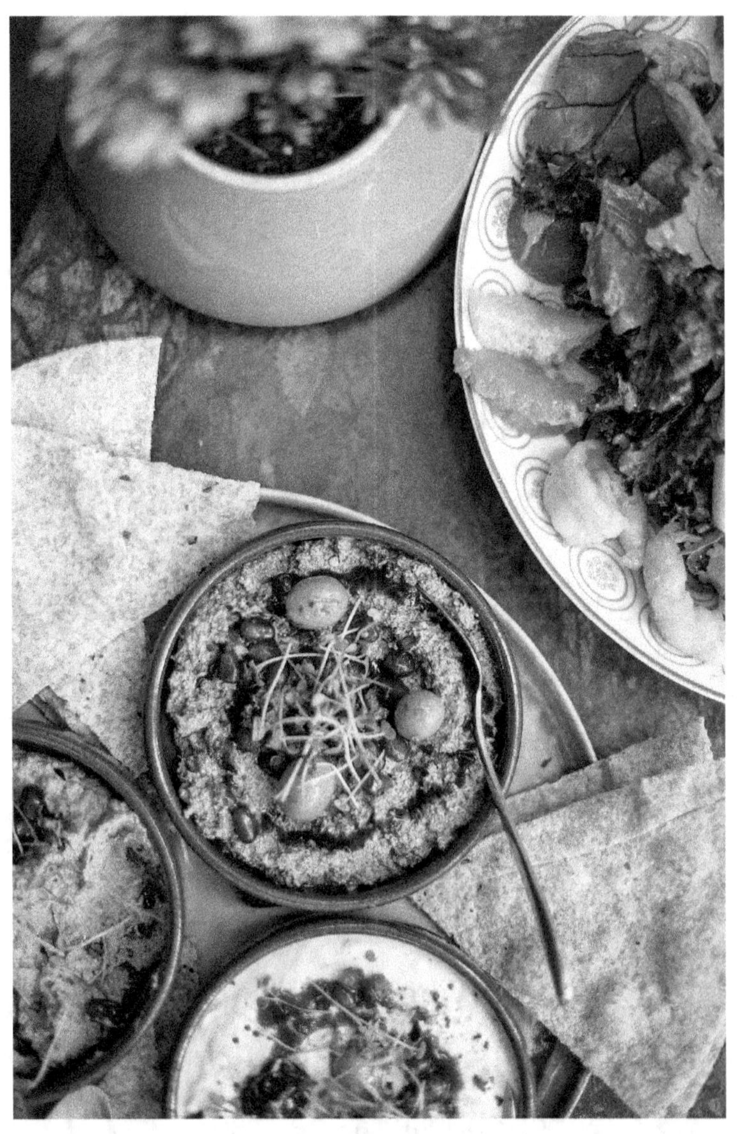

9. Spanish Tapas with Gazpacho Soup

A selection of Spanish tapas are served with a light and tasty lunch of cool gazpacho soup.

4 servings per item.

20 minutes are spent cooking and preparing.

Ingredients:

- 6 ripe tomatoes, diced, 1 cucumber, peeled and diced, 1 red bell pepper, diced, 1 small red onion, diced, 2 cloves of garlic, minced
- 3 glasses of tomato juice
- Red wine vinegar, 1/4 cup
- Olive oil, 1/4 cup
- pepper and salt as desired

- Various Spanish tapas, such as chorizo, Manchego cheese, and olives

Instructions:

1. The diced tomatoes, cucumber, red bell pepper, red onion, and minced garlic should all be combined in a blender.
2. Until smooth, blend.
3. Olive oil, red wine vinegar, and tomato juice should all be added to a blender. Remix the mixture until thoroughly blended.
4. Add salt and pepper to taste while preparing the gazpacho. Before serving, let the food cool for at least an hour in the refrigerator.

5. Along with a variety of Spanish tapas on the side, serve the gazpacho soup chilled.

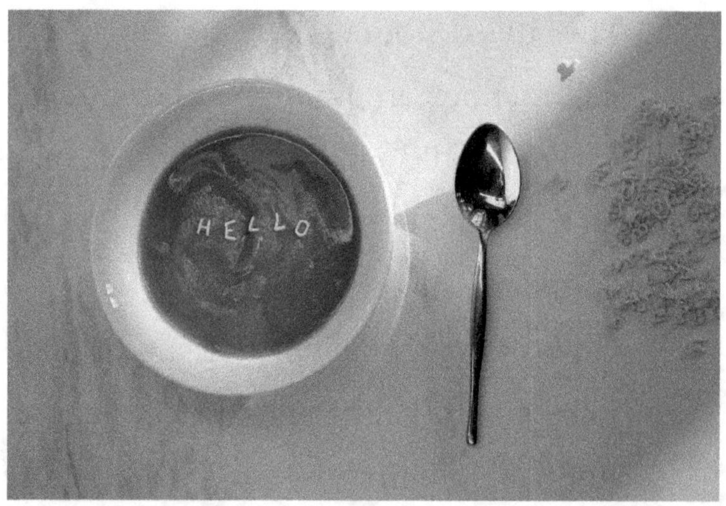

10. Teriyaki Tofu Skewers with Soba Noodle Soup

A delicious Asian-inspired supper including a hearty soba noodle soup and flavorful teriyaki tofu skewers.

4 servings per item.

Cooking and preparation time: 40 minutes

Ingredients:

- Soba noodles, 8 ounces
- 1 cup of sliced shiitake mushrooms in 4 cups of vegetable broth
- 1 serving baby spinach
- a serving of soy sauce
- 1 teaspoon of mirin
- 1/4 teaspoon ginger, grated
- pepper and salt as desired
- 1 brick of firm tofu, diced

- Teriyaki sauce to drizzle and use as a marinade
- Water-soaked wooden skewers

Instructions:

1. Soba noodles should be prepared as directed on the box. Drain, then set apart.

2. Bring vegetable broth to a boil in a big saucepan. Add baby spinach and thinly sliced shiitake mushrooms. Cook the mushrooms until they are soft.

3. Soy sauce, mirin, grated ginger, salt, and pepper are used to season the soup.

4. Tofu cubes should be marinated in teriyaki sauce for 15 minutes before being skewered with the sauce. They

should be grilled or baked until they have grill marks and are well cooked.

5. To serve, divide the cooked soba noodles into bowls and pour the mushroom and spinach-flavored hot broth over them. Teriyaki sauce should be drizzled over the tofu skewers.

6. Enjoy the teriyaki tofu skewers with the soba noodle soup.

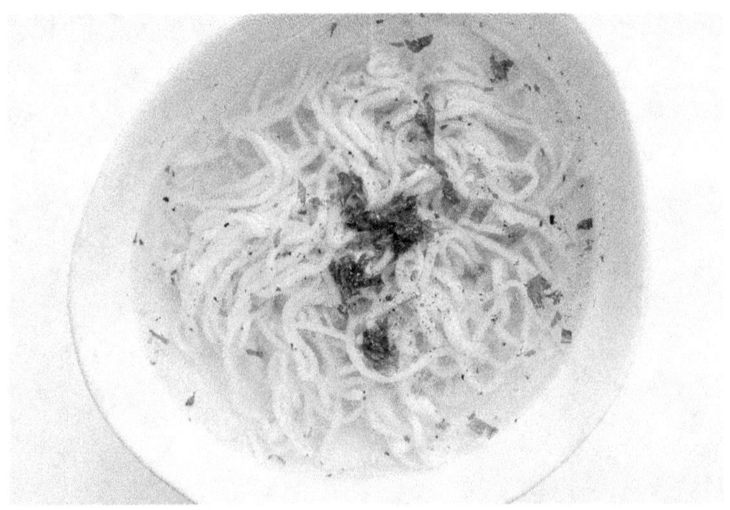

To accommodate different tastes and preferences, these recipes provide a wide variety of flavors and combinations. Take pleasure in your culinary explorations with these delicious soup and side dish pairings!

1. Peanut butter cups packed with protein

Brief Description/Background: These peanut butter cups are a guilt-free treat thanks to their high protein and low sugar content. They are a healthier version of a traditional favorite.

12 miniature glasses of serving size

20 minutes are spent cooking and preparing.

Ingredients:

- 1 cup natural, unsweetened peanut butter

- 1/four cup of chocolate or vanilla protein powder
- 1/4 cup maple syrup or honey
- a half-cup of 70% or more cacao dark chocolate chips
- Coconut oil, 1 tbsp
- as a garnish, sea salt

Step-by-step guidelines:

1. Mix the protein powder, honey/maple syrup, and peanut butter well in a bowl. Place aside.

2. Melt the dark chocolate chips and coconut oil in 30-second intervals in a microwave-safe bowl while stirring until smooth.

3. Use paper liners to line a tiny muffin tray. Each liner should have a thin layer of melted chocolate in the

bottom, which you should spread out evenly.

4. In each liner, top the chocolate with a little dollop of the peanut butter mixture.

5. Cover the peanut butter in each cup with the remaining melted chocolate.

6. On top of each cup, add a dash of sea salt.

7. Set in the refrigerator for at least an hour. Enjoy!

2. Protein Donuts with Baked Bananas

Brief Synopsis/Background Information: These baked banana protein donuts are a better option than regular fried donuts since they provide an increase in protein and a touch of natural sweetness from ripe bananas.

Size of Serving: 6 doughnuts

30-minute preparation and cooking time

Ingredients:

- 2 mashed ripe bananas
- 14 cups of vanilla protein powder
- Greek yogurt, 1/4 cup (unsweetened)
- 1/fourth cup almond milk
- 1 egg
- whole wheat flour, 1 cup
- one tablespoon of baking powder
- 1/four teaspoons of cinnamon
- A dash of salt
- Dark chocolate chips are optional as a garnish.

Step-by-step guidelines:

1. Set the oven's temperature to 350°F (175°C). Butter a doughnut pan.

2. Mash bananas, protein powder, Greek yogurt, almond milk, and egg in a bowl; combine ingredients well.

3. Combine whole wheat flour, baking soda, cinnamon, and salt in another basin.

4. Just enough liquid and dry components should be blended.

5. Fill each mold in the doughnut pan with approximately two-thirds of the batter.

6. The toothpick should come out clean after baking for 12 to 15 minutes.

7. After a brief period of cooling in the pan, remove the donuts and allow them to finish cooling on a wire rack.

8. For an extra treat, melt some dark chocolate chips and sprinkle them over the doughnuts.

3. Fresh Berry Chia Seed Pudding

Brief Synopsis/Background: This chia seed pudding is a tasty, healthy treat. Chia seeds, which are rich in fiber and omega-3 fatty acids, make a delightful and guilt-free treat when mixed with sweet, fresh berries.

Two servings per recipe

10 minutes for preparation and cooking (plus chilling time).

Ingredients:
- Chia seeds, 1/4 cup
- 1 cup of unsweetened almond milk
- 1 to 2 teaspoons of maple syrup or honey

- Vanilla extract, 1 teaspoon
- Topping of fresh mixed berries

Step-by-step guidelines:

1. Chia seeds, almond milk, honey or maple syrup, and vanilla essence should be combined in a bowl. To blend, thoroughly stir.

2. For the chia seeds to swell and take on the consistency of pudding, they must be covered and chilled for at least 2-3 hours or overnight.

3. Stir the ingredients before serving, then sprinkle the top with fresh mixed berries.

4. Avocado with Chocolate Mousse

Brief Synopsis/Background: Indulge in this luscious, creamy, avocado-based chocolate mousse. It offers healthy fats and rich tastes as an alternative to standard mousse.

4 servings per item.

Ten minutes for cooking and preparation

Ingredients:

- Two mature avocados
- cocoa powder, 1/4 cup
- 1/4 cup of agave nectar or honey
- Vanilla extract, 1 teaspoon
- A dash of salt
- Berries and shaved dark chocolate are optional garnishes.

Step-by-step guidelines:

1. Scoop the avocados out and put them in a food processor or blender.

2. Include vanilla essence, honey or agave syrup, cocoa powder, and a dash of salt.

3. Blend till creamy and smooth.

4. Distribute among serving glasses, then chill for at least 30 minutes.

5. Before serving, add berries or shaved dark chocolate as a garnish.

5. Cookies with Banana and Oats

Summary/History: Indulging in these banana oatmeal cookies won't make you feel bad. They are the ideal snack or dessert for anyone managing their sugar consumption since there is no added sugar to them.

Size of Serving: 12 cookies

20 minutes are spent cooking and preparing.

Ingredients:

- 2 mashed ripe bananas
- 1 Rolling oats, 1/2 cup
- One-half teaspoon of vanilla extract
- 14 cups finely chopped nuts, such as walnuts or almonds
- (Optional) 1/4 cup dark chocolate chips

Step-by-step guidelines:

1. Set the oven's temperature to 350°F (175°C). Use parchment paper to cover a baking sheet.
2. Bananas, rolled oats, vanilla essence, chopped almonds, and dark chocolate chips (if used) should all be well blended in a bowl.
3. Flattening the mixture slightly with the back of the spoon, drop spoonfuls

of the mixture onto the prepared baking sheet.

4. Until golden brown, bake for 12 to 15 minutes.

5. After a few minutes of cooling on the baking sheet, move the baked goods to a wire rack to finish cooling.

6. Fresh Berry and Greek Yogurt Parfait

This parfait is a delicious concoction of fresh berries, creamy Greek yogurt, and a drizzle of honey, making it a guilt-free and filling dessert or snack.

Size of Serving: 2 parfaits

Ten minutes for cooking and preparation

Ingredients:

- 1 cup of plain Greek yogurt

- Strawberries, blueberries, and raspberries make up one cup of mixed fresh berries.
- Honey, two tablespoons
- 14 cup optional granola for crunch

Step-by-step guidelines:

1. Greek yogurt and fresh berries should be layered in two serving glasses or bowls.
2. Honey should be drizzled on top.
3. Granola may be optionally added for taste and texture.
4. Serve right away and delight in it!

7. Chocolate-Covered Strawberries With Protein

Brief Synopsis/Background: These chocolate-covered strawberries satisfy your sweet tooth while also providing protein-rich enjoyment. They make a perfect romantic treat.

12 strawberries per serving

20 minutes are spent cooking and preparing.

Ingredients:

- big strawberries, twelve
- 12 cups of chocolate protein powder
- 14 cups of dark chocolate chips (at least 70% cocoa)
- Coconut oil, 1 tbsp

Step-by-step guidelines:

1. Thoroughly clean and dry the strawberries.

2. Create a thick paste in a bowl by combining the chocolate protein powder with a small quantity of water.

3. Each strawberry should be dipped into the protein paste and well-covered.

4. On a tray covered with parchment paper, place the coated strawberries, and freeze for 15 minutes.

5. Melt the dark chocolate chips and coconut oil in 30-second intervals in a microwave-safe bowl while stirring until smooth.

6. Each frozen strawberry should be dipped into the molten chocolate, allowing any extra to drop off.

7. Place the chocolate-coated strawberries back on the pan and put them in the fridge to let the chocolate set.

8. The protein-rich chocolate-covered strawberries are delicious!

8. Protein-rich banana bread

Brief Description/Background: This rendition of traditional banana bread is filled with protein and has the wholesome aromas of ripe bananas and almonds.

Size of Serving: 8 slices

1 hour for preparation and cooking

Ingredients:

- 2 mashed ripe bananas
- Vanilla protein powder, half a cup
- 14 cups almond meal
- chopped walnuts, 1/4 cup
- 1/4 cup maple syrup or honey
- 1 egg

- A half-teaspoon of baking soda

- half a teaspoon of cinnamon

- 14 teaspoons of salt

Step-by-step guidelines:

1. Set the oven's temperature to 350°F (175°C). Butter a loaf pan.

2. Bananas, protein powder, almond flour, walnuts, honey or maple syrup, eggs, baking soda, cinnamon, and salt should all be combined in a bowl.

3. Mix everything well until mixed.

4. Put the prepared loaf pan with the batter inside.

5. A toothpick inserted in the middle of the cake should come out clean after baking for 45 to 50 minutes.

6. Before moving the banana nut protein bread to a wire rack to finish cooling,

allow it to cool in the pan for 10 minutes.

9. Protein pancakes with blueberries

Brief Summary/Background: These light and fluffy blueberry protein pancakes are a delightful and invigorating way to start the day or fulfill your desires for pancakes guilt-free.

Servings per recipe: 2 (2-6 pancakes).

20 minutes are spent cooking and preparing.

Ingredients:

- rolled oats, 1 cup
- Vanilla protein powder, half a cup
- one ripe banana
- 50 ml of almond milk

- 1/2 cup blueberries, either fresh or frozen
- 1 egg
- one tablespoon of baking powder
- half a teaspoon of cinnamon
- A dash of salt
- Butter or cooking spray for the pan

Step-by-step guidelines:

1. Rollin oats, protein powder, ripe bananas, almond milk, blueberries, egg, baking soda, cinnamon, and a dash of salt should all be combined in a blender. Until smooth, blend.

2. Cooking spray or butter may be used to gently oil a non-stick pan or griddle before heating it.

3. To make pancakes, pour 1/4 cup sections of the batter onto the griddle.

4. Cook until surface bubbles appear, then turn and continue to cook until both sides are golden brown.

5. Continue by using the remaining batter.

6. If preferred, sprinkle your blueberry protein pancakes with honey or maple syrup before serving.

10. Chocolate Chia Seed Pudding

Brief Synopsis/Background: This chia seed chocolate pudding is a decadent and filling dessert that is high in protein and omega-3 fatty acids.

Two servings per recipe

5 minutes for preparation and cooking (plus chilling time).

Ingredients:

- Chia seeds, 1/4 cup

- almond milk, 1 cup

- Unsweetened cocoa powder, 2 teaspoons

- 2 teaspoons of maple syrup or honey

- One-half teaspoon of vanilla extract

- Optional garnishes: strawberries cut into slices, chopped almonds, or coconut flakes

Step-by-step guidelines:

1. Chia seeds, almond milk, chocolate powder, honey or maple syrup, and vanilla extract should all be combined in a bowl. Stir well to mix.

2. Stirring once or twice during this time will help avoid clumping. Cover the dish and place in the refrigerator for at least two hours or overnight.

3. Divide the mixture into serving plates after it has a pudding-like consistency and thickened.

4. If desired, garnish with shredded coconut, chopped almonds, or strawberry slices.

5. Offer cold.

These recipes provide a range of sweet delights that satisfy the sweet tooths of your health- and fitness-conscious audience while supporting their nutritional and health objectives. Enjoy!

Chapter 4

Managing Your Meal Balance: Portion Control and Macro Harmony

In this chapter, we examine the exacting science of attaining macronutrient harmony within each meal as well as the careful art of portion management. Learn how managing your macronutrient intake and knowing portion sizes may have a big influence on your quest for a leaner, stronger self.

Success in Bodybuilding: Portion Control

revealing the importance of portion control in calorie intake management.

Tips for managing and visualizing the right portion amounts for different food types.

Techniques for controlling your appetite without feeling restricted.

Achieving Macronutrient Equilibrium: The Macro-Puzzle

explaining the functions of the three macronutrients—carbohydrates, proteins, and fats—in your diet.

Guidelines for balancing your macronutrient intake to achieve your fitness goals.

How to balance your macronutrient intake for maximum energy, muscular development, and fat removal.

How to Create a Balanced Plate

Putting together a balanced dish with the proper proportions of proteins, veggies, carbohydrates, and healthy fats.

presenting well-balanced macronutrient examples for meals.

Changing portion control techniques to customize meals for different objectives, such as muscle building or weight reduction.

The Balance of Flavors: Improving Nutrition and Satisfaction

examining how eating well-balanced meals may satisfy both your appetite and your fitness objectives.

A few ideas for enhancing tastes and spices for a delicious meal without sacrificing nutrition.

promoting mindful eating with a well-rounded strategy.

You may make consistent progress toward your fitness goals by perfecting the art of portion management and the macronutrient balance in each meal. This chapter gives you the information and abilities to design your plate for the best outcomes, making sure that every bite you consume is in line with your objectives and leaves you feeling full and content.

Chapter 5

Investigating Cooking Methods for Healthier Foods

Cooking is an art, and learning the appropriate methods may change how you see food. Understanding and using the proper cooking techniques may go a long way toward creating healthier meals. This chapter takes us on a gastronomic adventure as we investigate cooking methods that not only improve taste but also put your health and well-being first.

1. **Grilling: Searing Excellence**

The pinnacle of healthful cooking is grilling. You may use it to give your foods an amazing taste without drenching them in oils or fats. The surface of veggies and lean meats caramelizes under the grill's intense, direct heat, producing that delectable char that gives your food depth. Grilling is a flexible cooking method that may give your healthy dishes new life, whether you're grilling veggies, lean pieces of meat, or even fruit.

2. Steaming Maintains Nutrients

The gentle giant of cooking techniques is steaming. It entails heating your foods over boiling water to preserve their original tastes and nutritional value. This method is ideal for individuals who want to save calories without sacrificing flavor. The vital vitamins and minerals are present in plenty in steamed veggies, seafood, and even dumplings.

3. Oven Magic: Baking and Roasting

When it comes to preparing the filling, healthful meals, baking and roasting are your friends. These cooking techniques produce meals with crisp textures and concentrated tastes by using dry heat in the oven. Your oven may serve as the foundation of your efforts to prepare nutritious meals, whether you're baking chicken breasts with a golden crust or roasting root vegetables with spices.

4. Quick and Colorful Sautéing and Stir-Frying

The cooking methods of sautéing and stir-frying stand out for their quickness and liveliness. They include frying little food items in little oil on a hot skillet. In addition to imparting a burst of flavor from herbs, spices, and aromatics, the fast cooking time preserves the natural crunch of vegetables and the suppleness of meats. These techniques are ideal for quickly producing foods that are nutrient-dense and vibrant.

5. Poaching: Gentle Elegance

Although poaching is a lesser-known technique, it is a valuable tool for making delicate, nutritious dishes. Food is poached when it is slowly simmered in a tasty liquid, usually water or broth. It's a technique that keeps meats, poultry, and shellfish unbelievably delicate while letting them take on the tastes of the food around them. Poached salmon, for example, is proof of the excellent outcomes possible with this method.

6. Blanking: The Door to Vibrant Colors
You can preserve the vivid colors and crisp textures of vegetables by blanching them. It entails quickly dipping components into icy water after submerging them in hot water. By stopping the cooking process, you may save your produce's nutrients and appealing appearance. Use blanched veggies as elegant sides or in salads and stir-fries.

You may improve your culinary skills and start down the path to improved health by learning how to make healthier meals. Each technique has its own special benefits that let you make a range of recipes that are both tasty and in line with your health objectives. So let's get our hands dirty, sharpen our knives, and embrace the art of cooking for a future that is both healthier and more delicious.

Methods to Cut Calories and Fat While Increasing Flavor:

Leaning toward a stronger, slimmer version of yourself does not mean giving up the pleasure of delectable meals. In reality, it is quite feasible to increase the taste of your food while lowering the amount of calories and fat in it. Here are some expert tips and useful methods to help you strike this precarious balance:

Conscious Ingredient Choice: Start by selecting lean proteins such as skinless chicken, fish, and lean beef cuts. Choose whole grains to improve fiber content and give you a sensation of fullness, including quinoa and brown rice.

Use cooking methods that need little additional oil, such as grilling, baking, steaming, and poaching. These techniques lower calorie consumption while maintaining the original aromas of the products.

Embrace a world of seasonings, herbs, and spices to improve your cuisine with flavorful spices and herbs. Try roasted vegetable recipes with garlic and rosemary or lean protein recipes with paprika and cumin. A simple dinner may become a culinary masterpiece with the addition of these ingredients.

Healthy Fats in Moderation: When cutting down on your consumption of fat, keep in mind that certain fats are necessary for taste. Sparingly use heart-healthy ingredients like olive oil, avocado, or almonds. To improve flavor, a little bit may go a long way.

Acidic Ingredients: You may add acidic and savory elements to your recipes without adding a lot of calories by using ingredients like vinegar, citrus juices, and low-sodium soy sauce. They work well for sauces and marinades.

Portion Control: It's important to get the hang of portion control. Smaller portions enable you to enjoy each meal while automatically lowering your calorie consumption. Use smaller plates to deceive your brain into thinking you need less food to feel full.

Examine healthy alternatives to reduce calories without sacrificing taste. To cut down on the amount of sugar and fat in your baked goods, swap out full-fat dairy with low-fat or Greek yogurt. You may also use applesauce or mashed bananas.

The Most Important Cooking Equipment for Your Fitness-Focused Culinary Journey:

You'll need the appropriate culinary equipment in your arsenal to successfully use these strategies. The following are the key cooking utensils to help you on your fitness-focused culinary journey:

Digital kitchen scale: Accurate calorie tracking and portion management depend on precise readings. You can be sure you're using the correct quantities of ingredients by utilizing a digital kitchen scale.

Quality Chef's Knife: Slicing and dicing are made easier and more fun by using a sharp chef's knife.

A steamer basket is ideal for cooking veggies since it helps preserve taste and nutrients while using fewer calories and fat.

Cookware that doesn't adhere to the pan: Non-stick pans use less oil, making them perfect for stir-frying and sautéing without adding too much fat.

Blender or food processor: These multipurpose appliances are necessary for making wholesome sauces, purees, and smoothies without additional fats.

Use a microplane grater to get the most flavor out of ingredients like ginger, garlic, and citrus zest without adding extra bulk.

Silicone baking mats: When baking low-fat sweets, these mats take the place of greasing pans and simplify cleaning.
Use an herb mill or mortar and pestle to grind fresh herbs and spices for meals that have strong, fragrant tastes.

This cooking equipment, together with the calorie and fat-cutting methods previously stated, will give you everything you need to create nourishing, delectable meals that support your fitness objectives without sacrificing taste. Here, at the center of your kitchen, is where your culinary journey to a leaner, stronger you starts.

Chapter 6

Your Individualized Meal Plans

Ready-Made Meal Plans for Various Fitness Objectives

Aligning your diet with your exercise objectives is one of the most important steps you can take on the road to a leaner, stronger self. This chapter goes into the core of your culinary journey and provides pre-made meal plans that have been painstakingly designed to meet different fitness goals. We offer a food plan that is specifically designed for you, whether your goals are weight reduction, muscle building, increased endurance, or just maintaining your present body.

1. Shred with Flavors: The Fat Loss Plan

Are you trying to get rid of extra weight and have a more toned body? Our fat loss program is designed to reduce calories while yet satisfying your cravings. Enjoy meals that were specifically chosen to promote fat loss, increase metabolism, and maintain energy levels.

2. Fuel Your Gains: The Muscle Building Blueprint

Our Muscle Building Blueprint offers the protein-rich, nutrient-dense meals necessary for muscle repair and development for people aiming to shape and strengthen their bodies. Learn about a variety of mouthwatering recipes that may help your body meet its demands for muscular growth.

3. Energize Your Workouts for Endurance Improvement

Our Endurance Enhancement plan is your ally if you're an athlete or fitness enthusiast looking to increase your stamina and endurance. During lengthy training or contests, these meals are intended to keep you functioning at your best while maximizing recuperation.

4. Live a Balanced Lifestyle and Continue to Succeed

Not all fitness journeys include radical changes. For those who have already made significant progress toward their objectives and want to keep it up, our Balanced Lifestyle meal plan is ideal. Enjoy delicious, well-balanced meals while allowing yourself occasional indulgences to promote your overall health.

5. Create Your Flexibility: Customize It

We are aware that each person's path to fitness is different. We provide recommendations and resources so you may adjust your meal plan to meet your unique requirements, tastes, and dietary restrictions. Make a strategy that is precisely in line with your lifestyle and fitness objectives.

Each meal plan in this chapter includes a comprehensive set of recipes, suggestions for serving sizes, and shopping lists. Our pre-made meal plans remove the worry from nutrition so you can enjoy the pleasure of consuming meals that will help you achieve your fitness goals, whether you're starting a new fitness journey or perfecting your current program.

Weekly meal plans for athletes, busy professionals, and more

Introduction:

Finding the time to make wholesome meals in today's hectic society may be difficult. This portion of the "Thinner Leaner Stronger Cookbook" is designed with your requirements in mind, whether you're a busy professional with a full schedule, an athlete aiming for top performance, or someone just trying to maintain a healthy lifestyle. We have designed weekly meal programs that promote convenience without sacrificing nutrition since we are aware of the responsibilities of your everyday life.

First mealtime: The Busy Workweek

This meal plan is intended to provide you with the energy you need throughout your tough workday.

4 servings per item.

30-minute preparation and cooking time

Ingredients:

- 1 pound of skinless, boneless chicken breasts
- quinoa, two cups
- 4 cups mixed veggies, including carrots, bell peppers, and broccoli
- Low-sodium soy sauce, 14 cup
- 2 minced garlic cloves
- Olive oil, 1 tbsp
- pepper and salt as desired

Instructions:

1. Quinoa should be prepared as directed on the packaging.

2. Chicken breasts should be salted and peppered.

3. Olive oil should be heated to a medium-high haze in a big skillet. Sauté for a minute after adding the minced garlic.

4. Add the chicken breasts and cook for 6 to 8 minutes on each side, or until browned. Take out and cut into strips.

5. Stir-fry mixed veggies in the same pan until they are soft.

6. Add the cooked quinoa and soy sauce to the pan with the chicken before heating through. Cook for a further 2–3 minutes after thoroughly stirring.

7. 4 servings should be served hot.

Second meal plan: athletes' power fuel

This meal plan offers the required nourishment for athletes wanting to maximize performance.

Two servings per recipe

Cooking and preparation time: 25 minutes

Ingredients:

- 1 serving brown rice
- 2 skinless, boneless filets of salmon
- Steamed broccoli, 2 cups
- 1 sliced lemon
- Olive oil, two teaspoons
- garnish with fresh dill
- pepper and salt as desired

Instructions:

1. Cook brown rice as directed on the box.
2. Olive oil, salt, and pepper are used to season salmon filets.
3. Grill salmon for four to five minutes on each side, or until it flakes easily.
4. Broccoli is steamed till soft.
5. With steamed broccoli lemon and fresh dill for garnish, plate grilled salmon over cooked brown rice.

Meal Plan #3: A Speedy and Filling Breakfast

Start your day off properly with this quick yet filling breakfast alternative.

Size of Serving: 1 serving

Ten minutes for cooking and preparation

Ingredients:

- Oats, rolled, in a cup
- 1 cup of almond milk without sugar
- 1 teaspoon of honey
- Fresh strawberries, blueberries, or raspberries, 1/4 cup
- 1 tablespoon of pecans, walnuts, or almonds that have been chopped

Instructions:

1. In a dish that can go in the microwave, combine almond milk and rolled oats.
2. Stirring every minute or so, heat the oats in the microwave on high for 2 to

3 minutes, or until the mixture thickens.

3. Add fresh berries and chopped almonds on top after drizzling honey over the dish.

4. Eat a short, wholesome breakfast.

Meal Plan #4: Quick Lunch Salad

A simple and wholesome salad for a hectic workday.

Size of Serving: 1 serving

15 minutes for cooking and preparation

Ingredients:

- 2 cups of mixed greens (kale, spinach, or arugula)
- Half a cup of cherry tomatoes
- Chickpeas, 1/4 cup, washed and drained
- sliced 1/4 cup of cucumber
- Balsamic vinaigrette, two teaspoons
- 2 tablespoons of feta cheese in crumbles
- pepper and salt as desired

Instructions:

1. Combine mixed greens, cherry tomatoes, chickpeas, and cucumber in a big bowl.

2. Add a balsamic vinaigrette drizzle and toss to coat.

3. Add salt & pepper and feta cheese crumbles as a garnish.

4. Enjoy a brief lunch that is cooling.

The fifth meal of the day is a protein smoothie.

A protein-rich smoothie to speed up recovery after a demanding exercise.

Size of Serving: 1 serving

Cooking and preparation time: 5 minutes

Ingredients:

- 1 cup of almond milk without sugar
- 1 scoop of protein powder in vanilla
- one ripe banana
- 1/4 cup almond butter
- half a teaspoon of cinnamon
- Ice cubes, if desired

Instructions:

1. Almond milk, protein powder, banana, almond butter, and cinnamon should all be combined in a blender.

2. If you would like a thicker texture, add ice cubes.

3. Once smooth, consume as a post-workout refuel.

Vegetarian Power Bowl is on the sixth day's menu.

A nutrient-rich dish for anyone choosing a vegetarian diet.

Two servings per recipe

30-minute preparation and cooking time

Ingredients:

- quinoa, one cup
- 1 can (15 oz) washed and drained black beans
- Roasted sweet potatoes, 1 cup
- 1 cup of spinach in sauce
- 1/4 cup red onion, chopped
- Olive oil, two teaspoons
- Balsamic vinegar, two teaspoons
- pepper and salt as desired

Instructions:

1. Quinoa should be prepared as directed on the packaging.
2. Black beans, roasted sweet potatoes, sautéed spinach, and sliced red onion are all combined in a dish.
3. drizzle with balsamic vinegar and olive oil. Add salt and pepper to taste.
4. The mixture should be served with cooked quinoa.

7th meal: Shrimp with Spicy Lemon and Garlic

An appetizing seafood meal ideal for a quick supper.

Two servings per recipe

20 minutes are spent cooking and preparing.

Ingredients:

- 8 ounces of big, peeled, and deveined shrimp
- 2 minced garlic cloves
- One lemon's juice and zest
- Olive oil, 1 tbsp
- garnishing with fresh parsley
- pepper and salt as desired

Instructions:

1. In a pan, heat the olive oil over medium-high heat. One minute after adding the minced garlic.

2. Add the shrimp and cook for two to three minutes on each side or until pink and opaque.

3. Lemon juice and zest should be drizzled over the dish, and salt and pepper should be added.

4. Serve hot and garnish with fresh parsley.

Meal Plan 8: A Boosting Breakfast Wrap

A breakfast sandwich filled with protein to get your day going.

Size of Serving: 1 serving

15 minutes for cooking and preparation

Ingredients:

- two huge eggs
- 2 tortillas made with whole wheat
- 14 cups of bell peppers, diced
- tomato dice, one-fourth cup
- 2 tablespoons of cheddar cheese, grated
- pepper and salt as desired
- Optional dipping sauce: salsa

Instructions:

1. In a pan, scramble eggs until they are fully cooked. Add salt and pepper to taste.

2. The whole wheat tortillas should be warmed for approximately 30 seconds on each side in the same pan.

3. Each tortilla should include scrambled eggs, diced bell peppers, diced tomatoes, and shredded cheddar cheese in the middle.

4. To add more flavor, roll up the tortillas and serve them with salsa.

Ninth meal: Nutty Yogurt Parfait

A filling yogurt parfait that makes a healthy snack or dessert.

Size of Serving: 1 serving

Ten minutes for cooking and preparation

Ingredients:

- Greek yogurt, one cup
- 1/4 cup of cereal
- Strawberries, blueberries, or raspberries make up 1/4 cup of the mixed fruit.
- 1 teaspoon of honey
- 1 tablespoon of pecans, walnuts, or almonds that have been chopped

Instructions:

1. Greek yogurt, granola, mixed berries, and honey should be arranged in a glass or dish.

2. For extra crunch and nutrients, sprinkle chopped nuts on top.

3. Enjoy as a filling dessert or snack.

High-Protein Veggie Stir-Fry, day 10 of the meal plan

A protein-rich stir-fry filled with vegetables for a speedy meal.

Two servings per recipe

20 minutes are spent cooking and preparing.

Ingredients:

- Bell peppers, broccoli, and snap peas make up two cups of the mixed veggies.
- Cubed 8 ounces of tofu, 2 teaspoons of low-sodium soy sauce
- one teaspoon of sesame oil
- 1 tablespoon ginger root, chopped
- 2 minced garlic cloves
- Green onions cut into 1/4 cup
- pepper and salt as desired

Instructions:

1. In a wok or large skillet, warm the sesame oil over medium-high heat.
2. Ginger and garlic that have been minced should be added.
3. Add the tofu and heat it until it is just beginning to brown.
4. Stir-fry the added mixed veggies for 4–5 minutes, or until they are soft.
5. Sprinkle with salt and pepper and drizzle with low-sodium soy sauce.
6. Serve hot and garnish with finely sliced green onions.

Grocery Lists to Make Your Preparations Simpler

Effective planning is essential before starting a path toward a healthier, slimmer, and stronger version of yourself. After planning your meals and setting your exercise objectives, it's time to go to the grocery store with a well-thought-out shopping list. Your secret weapon in the fight for culinary greatness and reaching your health goals is this plain old sheet of paper. Here are some reasons why and examples of how food shopping lists may make your preparations easier.

1. Simplifying the Shopping Process

Imagine entering a busy grocery shop without a list and being overwhelmed by the selection. Your concentration suddenly begins to wander, and you find yourself adding pointless products to your basket. This situation is all too typical, and it is exactly what a shopping list is meant to avoid.

You become a focused shopper when you have a list in order. You can quickly go around the shop since you are aware of precisely what you need and which aisles to go to. This not only saves you time but also helps you avoid making impulsive purchases that might interfere with your diet and exercise plans.

2. Ensuring Balanced Nutrition

Your grocery list serves as the basis for a well-balanced diet. It is a tool you may use to make sure you have everything you need to prepare meals that support your fitness goals. Whether it's a lean protein source, fresh veggies, or entire grains, every item on your list has a function.

You'll find it simpler to maintain the correct macronutrient balance and portion control if you stick to your list. It's a clear route to cooking meals that help you achieve your objectives, whether they're for general health, muscle building, or weight reduction.

3. Cutting down on food waste

Food waste reduction is one of the many advantages of a shopping list that is often disregarded. You're less likely to buy perishables that sit in your fridge when you just buy what you need for your scheduled meals. This helps to promote a more sustainable eating style while also saving you money.

4. Stress management

Making a list of things to buy in advance might be relaxing. It allows you to thoroughly analyze your meal plan and ensure that it is balanced and suited to your tastes. Before going to the supermarket, make sure you have everything you need to avoid last-minute stress and to feel confidently equipped to take on your culinary undertakings.

5. Individualization and Modification

Your grocery list is a very flexible tool. You may hone and customize your list as you gain more understanding of your dietary requirements and preferences. It alters as you go, taking into account advancements in your culinary and physical endeavors.

In conclusion, a well-organized grocery shopping list is your faithful ally on the road to a stronger, healthier version of yourself. It's a useful, time- and money-saving method that streamlines your preparations and guarantees you're always prepared to cook meals that support your fitness objectives. Make your shopping list now, before you go to the store. It's a modest effort that will pay out big on your path to greater health and energy.

Summary

Enjoying a Healthier You

The "Thinner Leaner Stronger Cookbook" has guided you on a tasty path to become a healthier and more powerful version of yourself. We have stressed the critical need to keep a balanced diet throughout these pages, not just as a temporary activity but as a lifetime commitment to your well-being.

Keep in mind that achieving health and fitness is a rewarding marathon, not a sprint. An investment in your long-term vitality is made with each meal you make from this cookbook, each dish you enjoy that is well-balanced, and each action you do to live a healthy lifestyle. Know that you are arming yourself with the information and skills to sculpt a healthier you as you continue to explore the varied and nutritious recipes, learn the art of meal planning, and use the professional techniques discussed within these pages. Your fitness path is characterized by tenacity, commitment, and the pleasure of consuming delicious, health-improving tastes.

So embrace this cookbook as your dependable ally as you pursue a better self. Let it be a reminder that the decisions you make now in your kitchen will influence the energy and vigor you experience in the years to come.

Let's toast to enjoying a healthy you, both now and for the rest of our lives.

Your One-Stop Resource Center

Knowledge is your most effective ally in your quest to become a healthier, slimmer, and stronger version of yourself. With the skills and knowledge you need to confidently manage your culinary and fitness journey, this thorough appendix serves as your go-to reference center.

1. Measurement guides and conversion tables

Getting the hang of cooking generally requires using exact measures. You may reliably follow our recipes exactly whether you're using metric or imperial units thanks to our conversion tables. No more speculating; simply flawless outcomes every time.

2. **Terms and Ingredients Glossary**

It's crucial to comprehend the language of nutrition and exercise. Our glossary translates the technical terms and introduces you to the essential components used in this recipe. We've got you covered when it comes to dietary terminology and intricate culinary skills.

3. **Additional Nutrition and Exercise Resources**

With this cookbook, your adventure doesn't come to an end; rather, it simply gets started. We've gathered several reliable sites for you to research more. With the help of books, websites, and professionals who can direct you on your route to success, delve further into the worlds of fitness, nutrition, and health.

The tools and knowledge in this appendix provide you the ability to make choices about your health and nutrition because, as they say, "knowledge is power."

Let this appendix be your dependable travel companion as you pursue your goal of becoming a healthier and more powerful version of yourself.

We appreciate your decision to buy the "Thinner Leaner Stronger Cookbook."

Here's to a bright future that is full of taste, health, and power!

Index

Meal Routines

Beginner's Manual

Sports Blueprint

Solution for Busy Professionals

N

Dinners Full of Nutrients

Salmon and chicken with asparagus and quinoa in a lemon-herb sauce vegetarian chili

O

P

Breakfasts Packed With Protein

Protein Pancakes with Oats

Breakfast Burrito with Spinach Feta and Greek Yogurt

Q

Simple & Quick Snacks

Greek cucumber cups, Nut Butter Banana Bites, Trail Mix Energy Bars

X

Y

Z

This thorough index makes it simple for readers to locate the knowledge they need to support their objectives for fitness and nutrition by giving rapid access to recipes and important subjects inside the cookbook.